INTRODUCTION

Metabolic confusion has emerged as a popular concept in the realm of diet and nutrition, promising to revolutionize weight loss and optimize metabolic function. Rooted in the belief that the human body can adapt to dietary patterns, metabolic confusion strategies aim to disrupt this adaptation process, leading to enhanced calorie burning and improved weight management outcomes. This approach suggests that by constantly varying aspects of one's diet, such as calorie intake, macronutrient composition, meal timing, and food choices, individuals can prevent their metabolism from settling into a stagnant state, thereby stimulating fat loss and metabolic efficiency.

Furthermore, dietary diversity is emphasized as a critical component of metabolic confusion, as it ensures that the body receives a broad spectrum of essential nutrients, micronutrients, and phytochemicals necessary for optimal metabolic function. This approach encourages individuals to incorporate a variety of whole foods, including fruits, vegetables, lean proteins, healthy fats, and complex carbohydrates, into their meal plans rather than relying on highly processed or restrictive dietary choices.

While metabolic confusion holds promise as a novel approach to weight management, its efficacy and long-term sustainability remain subjects of debate within the scientific community. Critics argue that the concept lacks robust empirical evidence and may promote unhealthy eating habits or unsustainable dietary practices.

CHAPTER ONE

Definition of Metabolic Confusion

Metabolic Confusion is a dietary strategy that aims to disrupt the body's adaptive responses to caloric intake and macronutrient composition, thereby purportedly enhancing metabolic rate and promoting weight loss. The concept revolves around the idea that the human body possesses a remarkable capacity to adapt to changes in energy balance, often leading to plateaus in weight loss and metabolic slowdown. By strategically varying aspects of one's diet, such as calorie intake, macronutrient ratios, meal timing, and food choices, metabolic Confusion seeks to prevent these adaptive responses and maintain metabolic flexibility.

CRITICAL COMPONENTS OF THE CONCEPT

• Caloric Variation: Metabolic Confusion involves alternating between caloric surplus and deficit periods rather than adhering to a consistent calorie intake. To keep the metabolism adaptable and responsive, this may include cycling between higher and lower calorie consumption days or implementing intermittent fasting protocols.

• Macronutrient Manipulation: Another core aspect of metabolic Confusion is the manipulation of macronutrient composition. This could involve varying the proportions of carbohydrates, proteins, and fats in the diet to prevent the body from adapting to a specific macronutrient profile and optimize metabolic function.

• Meal Timing: Meal timing is considered significant in metabolic Confusion, with proponents advocating for meal frequency and timing variations. These may include incorporating periodic fasting periods, adjusting meal timing throughout the day, or implementing strategies such as carb cycling to maximize metabolic flexibility.

• Dietary Diversity: Emphasizing dietary diversity is essential in metabolic Confusion to ensure that the body receives the nutrients necessary for optimal metabolic function. This involves incorporating a variety of whole foods, including fruits, vegetables, lean proteins, healthy fats, and complex carbohydrates, to support overall health and well-being.

HOW METABOLIC CONFUSION WORKS

Metabolic Confusion operates on the principle that the human body can adapt to changes in diet and energy expenditure. Traditional weight loss strategies often lead to plateaus as the body adjusts to reduced caloric intake, resulting in metabolic slowdown and diminished fat loss progress. Metabolic Confusion seeks to counteract these adaptations by constantly varying key dietary variables, thereby keeping the metabolism dynamic and responsive. Here's a comprehensive look at how metabolic Confusion works:

• Caloric Variation: Metabolic Confusion involves cycling between caloric surplus and deficit periods. By alternating between days of higher and lower calorie intake or implementing intermittent fasting protocols, metabolic Confusion prevents the body from settling into a predictable energy balance. This constant fluctuation in energy intake helps to keep the metabolism stimulated and prevents it from adjusting to a specific caloric level.

• Macronutrient Manipulation: Another crucial aspect of metabolic Confusion is manipulating macronutrient composition. This may include varying the proportions of carbohydrates, proteins, and fats in the diet. For example, individuals may alternate between high-carb and low-carb days or vary protein intake throughout the week. By constantly changing the macronutrient ratios, metabolic Confusion prevents the body from adapting to a specific nutrient profile, thereby enhancing fat loss and metabolic rate.

• Meal Timing: Meal timing is also an essential component of metabolic Confusion. Proponents of this approach advocate for variations in meal frequency and timing. This could involve incorporating periodic fasting periods, adjusting the timing of meals throughout the day, or implementing strategies such as carb cycling. By changing the timing of meals and nutrient intake, metabolic Confusion keeps the metabolism guessing and prevents it from settling into a routine.

• Dietary Diversity: Emphasizing dietary diversity is crucial in metabolic Confusion to ensure that the body receives a wide range of nutrients necessary for optimal metabolic function. This involves consuming a variety of whole foods, including fruits, vegetables, lean proteins, healthy fats, and complex carbohydrates. By incorporating diverse foods into the diet, metabolic Confusion supports overall health and well-being while preventing nutritional deficiencies.

• Adaptation Prevention: The primary goal of metabolic Confusion is to prevent the body from adapting to a specific caloric intake, macronutrient composition, or meal timing. By constantly changing these variables, metabolic Confusion keeps the metabolism flexible and responsive, leading to sustained fat loss and metabolic efficiency.

• Enhanced Metabolic Rate: By constantly challenging the body with diet and meal pattern variations, metabolic confusion propoConfusionue that the metabolic rate can be increased. This leads to more significant calorie expenditure and improved weight loss outcomes over time.

POTENTIAL BENEFITS OF THE METABOLIC CONFUSION DIET

The Metabolic Confusion diet has gained attention for its unique weight management and metabolic health approach. Advocates of this dietary strategy suggest that by constantly varying critical aspects of the diet, individuals can unlock a range of potential benefits that support overall well-being. The Metabolic Confusion diet offers several potential advantages:

Enhanced Metabolic Rate:

The constant fluctuations in caloric intake, macronutrient composition, and meal timing associated with the Metabolic Confusion diet may help to keep the metabolism stimulated and responsive. This can lead to an enhanced metabolic rate, resulting in more significant calorie expenditure and improved weight loss outcomes over time.

Prevention of Plateaus:

Traditional weight loss strategies often lead to plateaus as the body adapts to reduced caloric intake. Metabolic

Confusion may help prevent these plateaus by constantly changing critical aspects of the diet, allowing for more consistent progress toward weight loss goals.

Increased Fat Loss:

The variability in caloric intake, macronutrient composition, and meal timing associated with the Metabolic Confusion diet may promote more significant fat loss compared to traditional dieting approaches. By keeping the metabolism guessing and preventing adaptation, individuals may experience more substantial reductions in body fat over time.

Improved Metabolic Flexibility:

Metabolic ConfConfusionourages the body to become more flexible in its metabolic responses to dietary changes. By constantly challenging the metabolism with variations in diet and meal patterns, individuals may improve their metabolic flexibility, allowing for more efficient energy utilization and adaptation to different nutritional conditions.

Maintenance of Lean Muscle Mass:

Unlike traditional calorie-restricted diets, which may lead to muscle loss along with fat loss, the Metabolic Confusion diet aims to preserve lean muscle mass. By providing adequate protein intake and varying nutrient ratios, individuals can support muscle maintenance while promoting fat loss.

Psychological Benefits:

The flexibility and variety inherent in the Metabolic Confusion diet may offer psychological benefits compared to more restrictive dieting approaches. By allowing for occasional indulgences and variations in food choices, individuals may experience greater satisfaction and adherence to their dietary regimen.

Overall Health and Well-being:

The Metabolic Confusion diet promotes overall health and well-being by emphasizing dietary diversity and nutrient-rich foods. By incorporating a wide range of fruits, vegetables, lean proteins, healthy fats, and complex carbohydrates, individuals can ensure they receive the essential nutrients necessary for optimal metabolic function and overall health.

PRINCIPLES OF METABOLIC CONFUSION

The Metabolic Confusion approach to dieting revolves around strategic manipulation of key dietary variables to keep the body adaptable and responsive, thus promoting weight loss and metabolic efficiency. Here are the foundational principles of Metabolic Confusion:

A. Caloric Cycling:

• Low-Calorie Days:

• During low-calorie days, individuals consume fewer calories than their maintenance level. This creates a temporary calorie deficit, prompting the body to utilize stored fat for energy and facilitating weight loss. Low-calorie days are often interspersed throughout the week to prevent metabolic adaptation and promote fat burning.

• High-Calorie Days:

• On high-calorie days, individuals consume more calories than usual, typically at or slightly above their maintenance level. This temporarily increases energy intake, replenishes glycogen stores, and prevents metabolic slowdown. Thus, high-calorie days can help mitigate the negative effects of prolonged calorie restriction and support metabolic health.

B. Macronutrient Cycling:

• Low-Carb Days:

• Low-carb days restrict carbohydrate intake while emphasizing fat and protein intake. This approach promotes fat-burning and ketone production, as the body uses fats instead of carbohydrates as its primary fuel source. Low-carb days are commonly used to enhance fat loss and improve insulin sensitivity.

• High-Carb Days:

• Conversely, high-carb days involve increasing carbohydrate intake while moderating fat and protein intake. This replenishes glycogen stores, supports muscle recovery and performance, and provides a temporary metabolic boost. High-carb days can help to prevent metabolic adaptation, maintain metabolic flexibility, and enhance exercise performance.

C. Meal Timing and Frequency:

• Intermittent Fasting Options:

• Intermittent fasting involves cycling between periods of eating and fasting, typically daily or weekly. Standard protocols include the 16/8 method (fasting for 16 hours and eating within an 8-hour window), alternate-day fasting, and periodic fasting. Intermittent fasting promotes fat loss, improves metabolic health, and enhances cellular repair processes.

• Meal Spacing Strategies:

• Meal spacing refers to the timing and frequency of meals throughout the day. Strategies may include consuming smaller, more frequent meals or practicing longer intervals between meals. By manipulating meal timing and frequency, individuals can optimize nutrient partitioning, control hunger and satiety, and support metabolic flexibility. Meal spacing strategies may complement intermittent fasting protocols to enhance metabolic outcomes.

IMPLEMENTING THE METABOLIC CONFUSION DIET

The Metabolic Confusion diet offers a flexible and dynamic weight management and metabolic health approach. Here's a comprehensive guide on how to implement this dietary strategy:

A. Initial Assessment and Goal Setting:

• Evaluation of Current Health Status:

• Before starting the Metabolic Confusion diet, you must assess your current health status, including any medical conditions, dietary preferences, and lifestyle factors. Consider consulting with a healthcare professional or registered dietitian to ensure the approach suits your needs.

• Setting Realistic Goals for Weight Loss or Body Composition Changes:

• Establish realistic and achievable goals for weight loss, fat loss, or body composition changes based on your personal objectives and timeframe. Focus on setting specific, measurable, attainable, relevant, and time-bound (SMART) goals to guide your progress and keep you motivated.

B. Calorie and Macronutrient Calculation:

• Determining Daily Caloric Needs:

• Calculate your estimated daily caloric needs based on factors such as age, gender, weight, height, activity level, and goals. Use online calculators or consult with a healthcare professional to determine your baseline calorie requirements.

• Macronutrient Ratios for Different Days:

• Determine the macronutrient ratios for low-calorie and high-calorie days based on your goals and preferences. For example, low-calorie days may involve higher protein and fat intake with moderate carbohydrate consumption. In contrast, high-calorie days may include higher carbohydrate intake with moderate protein and fat consumption.

C. Meal Planning and Food Choices:

• Designing Meals for Low-Calorie and High-Calorie Days:

• Plan your meals and snacks in advance, taking into account each day's calorie and macronutrient targets. Focus on incorporating nutrient-dense foods such as lean proteins, fruits, vegetables, whole grains, and healthy fats to support overall health and satiety.

• Selecting Nutrient-Dense Foods:

• Choose nutrient-dense foods that provide essential vitamins, minerals, and antioxidants while supporting your calorie and macronutrient goals. Avoid highly processed foods, sugary snacks, and empty calories, opting instead for whole, minimally processed options.

D. Rotation Schedule:

• Establishing a Cycling Pattern (e.g., Weekly or Biweekly):

• Develop a rotation schedule that alternates between low-calorie and high-calorie days, as well as varying macronutrient ratios and meal timing. Depending on your preferences and goals, this may involve cycling on a weekly or biweekly basis.

• Monitoring and Adjusting Based on Progress:

• Monitor your progress regularly, including changes in weight, body composition, energy levels, and overall well-being. Adjust your calorie and macronutrient intake, meal planning, and rotation schedule as needed based on your progress and body feedback.

E. Exercise Integration:

• Tailoring Exercise to Caloric Intake:

• Adapt your exercise routine to align with your caloric intake and energy needs on different days. Consider focusing on strength training and resistance exercises on high-calorie days to support muscle growth and recovery. On low-calorie days, prioritize cardiovascular activities and endurance training to maximize calorie burning and fat loss.

• Combining Cardiovascular and Strength Training:

• To promote overall fitness and metabolic health, incorporate a combination of cardiovascular exercise, such as running, cycling, or swimming, with strength training exercises, such as weightlifting or bodyweight exercises. Aim for a balanced exercise regimen that includes both aerobic and anaerobic activities.

F. Hydration and Supplementation:

- Importance of Hydration in Metabolism:

- Drink adequate water throughout the day, especially during periods of increased physical activity or calorie restriction. Proper hydration supports metabolism, regulates appetite and promotes overall health and well-being.

- Consideration of Supplements for Nutritional Support:

- Consider incorporating dietary supplements, such as vitamins, minerals, and herbal extracts, to support your nutritional needs and optimize metabolic function. Consult with a healthcare professional or registered dietitian to determine if supplementation is appropriate for you based on your individual requirements and goals.

TRACKING AND MONITORING PROGRESS

Tracking and monitoring progress are essential components of any successful dietary and fitness regimen, including the Metabolic Confusion diet. Here's a comprehensive guide on how to effectively track and monitor your progress:

A. Measurement Tools:

• Weighing Scale:

• The weighing scale is a fundamental tool for tracking changes in body weight over time. Regular weigh-ins, preferably under consistent conditions (e.g., exact time of day, same clothing), can provide valuable insights into your progress and help you adjust your dietary and exercise strategies accordingly.

• Body Composition Analysis (e.g., Body Fat Percentage):

• Body composition analysis provides a more comprehensive assessment of your progress beyond just body weight. Methods such as bioelectrical impedance analysis (BIA), skinfold calipers, or dual-energy X-ray absorptiometry (DEXA) can help you track changes in body fat percentage, lean muscle mass, and overall body composition.

B. Tracking Methods:

• Food Journaling:

• Keeping a detailed food journal allows you to monitor your daily dietary intake, including calorie consumption, macronutrient breakdown, and meal timing. Recording your meals and snacks can help you identify patterns, track progress toward your nutritional goals, and make informed adjustments to your diet as needed.

• Exercise Logs:

• Maintaining an exercise log enables you to track your physical activity levels, workout frequency, intensity, and duration. Whether it's strength training sessions, cardiovascular exercise, or other forms of physical activity, logging your workouts allows you to monitor progress, identify areas for improvement, and ensure consistency in your exercise routine.

C. Assessing Results and Adjustments:

• Analyzing Changes in Weight and Body Composition:

• Regularly assess changes in body weight, body fat percentage, and other relevant metrics to gauge your progress on the Metabolic Confusion diet. Compare measurements over time to identify trends and patterns, such as weight fluctuations or body composition improvements. Remember that progress may not always be linear, and minor fluctuations are normal.

• Modifying Diet and Exercise Plans as Needed:

• Based on your progress assessment and feedback from tracking tools, make informed adjustments to your diet and exercise plans as needed. If you're not seeing the desired results, consider adjusting your calorie intake, macronutrient ratios, meal timing, or exercise regimen. Be flexible and willing to experiment with different strategies to optimize your outcomes.

LONG-TERM SUSTAINABILITY AND MAINTENANCE

Achieving long-term success with any dietary plan, including the Metabolic Confusion approach, requires a sustainable lifestyle approach and ongoing maintenance strategies. Here's a comprehensive guide on how to ensure the sustainability of your progress and maintain your results over the long term:

A. Lifestyle Integration:

• Incorporating Healthy Habits Beyond the Diet Plan:

• Sustainable success on the Metabolic Confusion diet involves more than just following a specific eating regimen. It requires integrating healthy habits into your lifestyle, such as regular physical activity, stress management techniques, adequate hydration, and mindfulness practices. Focus on creating a balanced lifestyle that supports your overall well-being beyond diet and exercise alone.

• Stress Management and Sleep Optimization:

• Stress management and quality sleep are essential components of long-term health and weight management. Practice stress-reducing activities such as meditation, yoga, deep breathing exercises, or spending time outdoors. Prioritize adequate sleep hygiene habits, aiming for 7-9 hours of quality sleep per night to support optimal metabolic function and overall health.

B. Transitioning to Maintenance Phase:

• Gradual Adjustment of Caloric Intake:

• As you progress with the Metabolic Confusion diet and reach your desired weight or body composition goals, gradually transition to a maintenance phase by adjusting your caloric intake accordingly. Gradually increase your calorie intake to match your energy expenditure and support weight maintenance while avoiding rapid weight regain.

• Focus on Sustainable Eating Patterns:

• Shift your focus from strict calorie counting and macro cycling to adopting sustainable eating patterns that promote overall health and well-being. Emphasize nutrient-dense whole foods, balanced meals, and intuitive eating practices that support long-term dietary adherence and enjoyment.

C. Support and Accountability:

• Seeking Support from Peers or Professionals:

• Surround yourself with a supportive network of friends, family, or health professionals who can encourage, hold you accountable, and guide you throughout your journey. To stay motivated and accountable, consider joining online communities, support groups or working with a registered dietitian or fitness coach.

• Celebrating Achievements and Overcoming Challenges:

• Celebrate your achievements, no matter how small,

and acknowledge your progress along the way. Recognize the challenges you've overcome and the obstacles you've faced with resilience and determination. Use setbacks as learning opportunities to refine your approach and continue moving forward towards your long-term goals.

CHAPTER TWO

Low-Calorie Recipes

Grilled Chicken Salad with Mixed Greens
and Balsamic Vinaigrette

Meal Description: This Grilled Chicken Salad with Mixed Greens and Balsamic Vinaigrette is a light and satisfying meal that's perfect for lunch or dinner. Tender grilled chicken breast is served atop a bed of fresh mixed greens, cherry tomatoes, cucumber slices, and red onion, then drizzled with a tangy balsamic vinaigrette. Packed with flavor and nutrients, this salad is delicious and nutritious, making it an ideal choice for those seeking a healthy and satisfying meal.

Ingredients:

• 4 oz boneless, skinless chicken breast

• 4 cups mixed salad greens (such as lettuce, spinach, arugula)

• 1/2 cup cherry tomatoes, halved

• 1/4 cup cucumber, sliced

• 1/4 cup red onion, thinly sliced

• 2 tbsp balsamic vinegar

• 1 tbsp olive oil

• 1 tsp Dijon mustard

• Salt and pepper to taste

Instructions:

1. Preheat the grill or grill pan to medium-high heat.

2. Season the chicken breast with salt and pepper on both sides.

3. Place the chicken breast on the grill and cook for 6-8 minutes per side or until cooked through and no longer pink in the center. Remove from heat and let rest for a few minutes before slicing.

4. To make the vinaigrette, whisk together balsamic vinegar, olive oil, Dijon mustard, salt, and pepper in a small bowl.

5. Combine mixed salad greens, cherry tomatoes, cucumber slices, and red onion in a large mixing bowl.

6. Divide the salad mixture evenly between two plates.

7. Slice the grilled chicken breast and arrange on top of each salad.

8. Drizzle the balsamic vinaigrette over the salads.

9. Serve immediately and enjoy!

Nutrition Information (per serving):

• Calories: 230

• Protein: 24g

• Fat: 10g

• Carbohydrates: 10g

• Fiber: 3g

• Sugar: 5g

• Sodium: 350mg

VEGETABLE STIR-FRY WITH TOFU AND SOY SAUCE

Meal Description: This Vegetable Stir-Fry with Tofu and Soy Sauce is a flavorful and nutritious dish that's perfect for a quick and easy weeknight dinner. It features a colorful assortment of fresh vegetables, including bell peppers, broccoli, carrots, and snap peas, stir-fried with crispy tofu, and seasoned with a savory soy sauce-based sauce. Serve this delicious stir-fry over steamed rice or noodles for a satisfying meal that's packed with plant-based protein and vibrant flavors.

Ingredients:

- 14 oz extra-firm tofu, pressed and cubed
- 2 cups mixed vegetables (bell peppers, broccoli florets, carrots, snap peas)
- Two cloves garlic, minced
- 2 tbsp soy sauce (low-sodium if preferred)
- 1 tbsp sesame oil
- 1 tbsp cornstarch
- 1 tbsp vegetable oil

- 1 tsp grated ginger

- Optional toppings: sliced green onions, sesame seeds

Instructions:

1. To remove excess moisture, press the tofu between paper towels or use a tofu press. Cut the tofu into bite-sized cubes and set aside.

2. To make the sauce, whisk together soy sauce, sesame oil, cornstarch, minced garlic, and grated ginger in a small bowl. Set aside.

3. Heat vegetable oil in a large skillet or wok over medium-high heat. Add the cubed tofu and cook until golden and crispy on all sides, about 5-7 minutes. Remove tofu from the skillet and set aside.

4. Add a bit more oil, if needed, in the same skillet, then add the mixed vegetables. Stir-fry for 4-5 minutes or until the vegetables are tender-crisp.

5. Return the cooked tofu to the skillet with the vegetables.

6. Pour the prepared sauce over the tofu and vegetables. Stir well to coat everything evenly in the sauce.

7. Cook for an additional 2-3 minutes or until the sauce has thickened and everything is heated through.

8. Remove from heat and immediately serve the Vegetable Stir-Fry with Tofu and Soy Sauce, garnished with sliced green onions and sesame seeds if desired.

9. Enjoy this delicious and nutritious dish served over steamed rice or noodles!

Nutrition Information (per serving):

- Calories: 250

- Protein: 18g
- Fat: 14g
- Carbohydrates: 16g
- Fiber: 4g
- Sugar: 4g
- Sodium: 480mg

ZUCCHINI NOODLES (ZOODLES) WITH MARINARA SAUCE AND TURKEY MEATBALLS

Meal Description: Indulge in a healthier twist on classic comfort food with these Zucchini Noodles (Zoodles) with Marinara Sauce and Turkey Meatballs. This wholesome dish features zucchini noodles, also known as zoodles, tossed in a flavorful marinara sauce and topped with lean turkey meatballs. Packed with veggies and protein, this low-carb and gluten-free meal is satisfying, delicious, and perfect for those seeking a lighter alternative to traditional pasta dishes.

Ingredients:

For Turkey Meatballs:

• 1 lb lean ground turkey

• 1/4 cup breadcrumbs (gluten-free if preferred)

- 1/4 cup grated Parmesan cheese
- One egg
- Two cloves garlic, minced
- 1 tsp Italian seasoning
- Salt and pepper to taste
- 1 tbsp olive oil (for cooking)

For Zucchini Noodles and Marinara Sauce:

- Four medium zucchini spiralized into noodles
- 2 cups marinara sauce (store-bought or homemade)
- 1 tbsp olive oil
- Two cloves garlic, minced
- Salt and pepper to taste
- Fresh basil leaves for garnish
- Grated Parmesan cheese for serving (optional)

Instructions:

1. Prepare Turkey Meatballs:

- Combine ground turkey, breadcrumbs, grated Parmesan cheese, egg, minced garlic, Italian seasoning, salt, and pepper in a large mixing bowl. Mix until well combined.

- Shape the mixture into meatballs about 1 inch in diameter.

- Heat olive oil in a large skillet over medium heat. Add the turkey meatballs and cook until browned on all sides, about 10-12 minutes. Remove from heat and set aside.

1. Prepare Zucchini Noodles and Marinara Sauce:

- In the same skillet, heat olive oil over medium heat. Add

minced garlic and cook for 1-2 minutes, until fragrant.

• Add the spiralized zucchini noodles to the skillet and sauté for 3-4 minutes, until tender but still slightly crisp.

• Pour marinara sauce over the zucchini noodles and stir to combine. Cook for an additional 2-3 minutes until heated through.

1. Assemble and Serve:

• Divide the zucchini noodles and marinara sauce among serving plates.

• Top each plate with turkey meatballs.

• Garnish with fresh basil leaves and grated Parmesan cheese, if desired.

1. Enjoy your Zucchini Noodles with Marinara Sauce and Turkey Meatballs!

Nutrition Information (per serving):

• Calories: 290

• Protein: 27g

• Fat: 12g

• Carbohydrates: 18g

• Fiber: 4g

• Sugar: 8g

• Sodium: 670mg

EGG WHITE OMELETTE WITH SPINACH, MUSHROOMS, AND TOMATOES

Meal Description: Start your day on a nutritious note with this Egg White Omelette with Spinach, Mushrooms, and Tomatoes. This protein-packed breakfast is light, flavorful, and bursting with colorful vegetables. Egg whites are cooked to perfection and filled with sautéed spinach, mushrooms, and tomatoes for a satisfying and wholesome morning meal.

Ingredients:

- Six egg whites

- 1 cup fresh spinach leaves, chopped

- 1/2 cup mushrooms, sliced

- 1/2 cup cherry tomatoes, halved

- 1/4 cup onion, finely chopped

- One clove of garlic, minced

• 1 tsp olive oil

• Salt and pepper to taste

• Optional: grated cheese for topping

Instructions:

1. Prepare Vegetables:

• Heat olive oil in a non-stick skillet over medium heat.

• Add minced garlic and chopped onion to the skillet and sauté for 2-3 minutes, until fragrant.

• Add sliced mushrooms to the skillet and cook for 4-5 minutes, until softened.

• Add chopped spinach leaves and halved cherry tomatoes to the skillet. Cook for an additional 2-3 minutes, until spinach is wilted and tomatoes are softened. Season with salt and pepper to taste. Remove vegetables from the skillet and set aside.

1. Cook Egg Whites:

• In a separate bowl, whisk egg whites until frothy.

• Pour the whisked egg whites into the same skillet used for the vegetables, spreading them evenly to cover the bottom of the skillet.

• Cook the egg whites for 2-3 minutes or until the edges begin to set.

1. Assemble Omelette:

• Once the egg whites are partially cooked, spoon the cooked vegetables onto one-half of the omelet.

• Gently fold the other half of the omelet over the vegetables, forming a half-moon shape.

• Cook for an additional 1-2 minutes, until the omelet is

cooked through and slightly golden on the outside.

1. Serve:

• Carefully transfer the omelette to a plate.

• If desired, sprinkle grated cheese over the top of the omelet.

• Serve hot, and enjoy your Egg White Omelette with Spinach, Mushrooms, and Tomatoes!

Nutrition Information (per serving):

• Calories: 120

• Protein: 20g

• Fat: 3g

• Carbohydrates: 5g

• Fiber: 2g

• Sugar: 2g

• Sodium: 290mg

CUCUMBER AND TOMATO SALAD WITH LEMON-HERB DRESSING

Meal Description: This refreshing Cucumber and Tomato Salad with Lemon-Herb Dressing is a light, vibrant side dish that complements any meal. Crisp cucumber slices and juicy cherry tomatoes are tossed in a zesty lemon-herb dressing, creating a perfect balance of flavors. This salad is quick to prepare and bursting with fresh ingredients, making it an ideal accompaniment to any summer barbecue or dinner spread.

Ingredients:

For Salad:

• Two large cucumbers, thinly sliced

• 1 pint cherry tomatoes, halved

• 1/4 cup red onion, thinly sliced

• 2 tbsp fresh parsley, chopped

• Salt and pepper to taste

For Lemon-Herb Dressing:

- 3 tbsp olive oil
- 2 tbsp fresh lemon juice
- 1 tsp lemon zest
- 1 tsp honey or maple syrup (optional)
- One clove of garlic, minced
- 1 tbsp fresh basil, chopped
- 1 tbsp fresh mint, chopped
- Salt and pepper to taste

Instructions:

1. Prepare Salad Ingredients:

- Combine thinly sliced cucumbers, halved cherry tomatoes, thinly sliced red onion, and chopped fresh parsley in a large mixing bowl. Season with salt and pepper to taste. Set aside.

1. Prepare Lemon-Herb Dressing:

- In a small bowl, whisk together olive oil, fresh lemon juice, lemon zest, honey or maple syrup (if using), minced garlic, chopped fresh basil, and chopped fresh mint. Season with salt and pepper to taste. Adjust the sweetness and acidity according to your preference.

1. Assemble Salad:

- Pour the prepared lemon-herb dressing over the cucumber and tomato mixture into a large mixing bowl.

- Gently toss the salad until all ingredients are evenly coated with the dressing.

1. Chill and Serve:

- Cover the salad and refrigerate for at least 30 minutes to allow the flavors to meld together.

• Before serving, give the salad a final toss to redistribute the dressing.

• Garnish with additional fresh herbs if desired.

1. Enjoy your Cucumber and Tomato Salad with Lemon-Herb Dressing!

Nutrition Information (per serving):

• Calories: 80

• Protein: 2g

• Fat: 6g

• Carbohydrates: 7g

• Fiber: 2g

• Sugar: 4g

• Sodium: 15mg

STEAMED FISH WITH BROCCOLI AND QUINOA

Meal Description: This Steamed Fish with Broccoli and Quinoa is a nutritious and balanced meal that's simple to prepare and bursting with flavor. Tender fish fillets are steamed to perfection and served alongside steamed broccoli florets and fluffy quinoa. This dish is delicious and packed with protein, fiber, vitamins, and minerals, making it an ideal choice for a wholesome dinner.

Ingredients:

For Steamed Fish:

- Four fish fillets (such as tilapia, salmon, or cod)

- Salt and pepper to taste

- Lemon slices for garnish (optional)

For Steamed Broccoli:

- 2 cups broccoli florets

- 1 tbsp olive oil

- Salt and pepper to taste

For Quinoa:

- 1 cup quinoa, rinsed

• 2 cups water or vegetable broth

• Salt to taste

Instructions:

1. Prepare Quinoa:

• In a saucepan, combine rinsed quinoa and water or vegetable broth. Bring to a boil over medium-high heat.

• Reduce heat to low, cover, and simmer for 15-20 minutes until quinoa is tender and water is absorbed.

• Remove from heat and cover the quinoa for 5 minutes. Fluff with a fork and season with salt to taste.

1. Prepare Steamed Broccoli:

• While the quinoa is cooking, steam the broccoli florets until tender-crisp. You can use a steamer basket over boiling water or in the microwave.

• Once steamed, toss the broccoli with olive oil, salt, and pepper to taste.

1. Prepare Steamed Fish:

• Season fish fillets with salt and pepper to taste.

• Place fish fillets in a single layer in a steamer basket or on a plate suitable for steaming.

• Steam the fish fillets for 8-10 minutes until they are cooked through and flake easily with a fork.

1. Assemble and Serve:

• Divide the cooked quinoa, steamed broccoli, and steamed fish fillets among serving plates.

• Garnish with lemon slices if desired.

• Serve immediately, and enjoy your Steamed Fish with

Broccoli and Quinoa!

Nutrition Information (per serving):

- Calories: 300

- Protein: 25g

- Fat: 8g

- Carbohydrates: 30g

- Fiber: 6g

- Sugar: 2g

- Sodium: 200mg

TURKEY AND VEGGIE LETTUCE WRAPS WITH HUMMUS

Meal Description: These Turkey and Veggie Lettuce Wraps with Hummus are a light, refreshing, and flavorful meal option that's perfect for a quick lunch or dinner. Crisp lettuce leaves are filled with seasoned ground turkey, colorful vegetables, and creamy hummus, creating a satisfying and nutritious meal that's low in carbs and high in protein. Enjoy these lettuce wraps as a healthy and delicious alternative to traditional sandwiches or wraps.

Ingredients:

For Turkey Filling:

- 1 lb lean ground turkey

- 1 tbsp olive oil

- 1/2 onion, diced

- Two cloves garlic, minced

- One bell pepper, diced

- OneOne zucchini, diced
- OneOne carrots, grated
- 1 tsp ground cumin
- 1 tsp chili powder
- Salt and pepper to taste

For Lettuce Wraps:

- Large lettuce leaves (such as romaine or butter lettuce)
- Hummus (store-bought or homemade)

Optional Toppings:

- Cherry tomatoes, halved
- Cucumber slices
- Avocado slices
- Fresh cilantro leaves
- Lime wedges

Instructions:

1. Prepare Turkey Filling:

- Heat olive oil in a large skillet over medium heat.

- Add diced onion and minced garlic to the skillet and sauté for 2-3 minutes, until fragrant.

- Add ground turkey to the skillet and cook until browned, breaking it up with a spoon as it cooks.

- Stir in diced bell pepper, diced zucchini, grated carrot, ground cumin, chili powder, salt, and pepper. Cook for an additional 5-6 minutes, until vegetables are tender and turkey is cooked through.

1. Assemble Lettuce Wraps:

• Spoon a portion of the turkey and veggie filling onto each lettuce leaf.

• Spread a dollop of hummus over the filling.

• If desired, add optional toppings such as cherry tomatoes, cucumber slices, avocado slices, fresh cilantro leaves, and a squeeze of lime juice.

1. Serve:

• Roll up the lettuce leaves to enclose the filling, securing them with toothpicks if necessary.

• Arrange the lettuce wraps on a serving platter and serve immediately.

1. Enjoy your Turkey and Veggie Lettuce Wraps with Hummus!

Nutrition Information (per serving - 2 lettuce wraps):

• Calories: 250

• Protein: 25g

• Fat: 12g

• Carbohydrates: 10g

• Fiber: 4g

• Sugar: 3g

• Sodium: 350mg

SHRIMP AND VEGETABLE SKEWERS WITH LEMON-GARLIC MARINADE

Meal Description: Delight your taste buds with these Shrimp and Vegetable Skewers marinated in a zesty Lemon-garlic marinade. Succulent shrimp, colorful bell peppers, cherry tomatoes, and zucchini come together on skewers, creating a vibrant and flavorful dish. Grilled to perfection, these skewers are perfect for a light and refreshing meal, showcasing the natural flavors of the ingredients enhanced by the bright and citrusy marinade.

Ingredients:

For Lemon-Garlic Marinade:

• 1/4 cup olive oil

• 3 tbsp fresh lemon juice

• Two cloves garlic, minced

• 1 tsp lemon zest

- 1 tsp honey or maple syrup

- 1 tsp dried oregano

- Salt and pepper to taste

For Shrimp and Vegetable Skewers:

- 1 lb large shrimp, peeled and deveined

- One red bell pepper, cut into chunks

- One yellow bell pepper, cut into chunks

- One zucchini, sliced into rounds

- Cherry tomatoes

- Wooden or metal skewers (pre-soak wooden skewers in water for 30 minutes if using)

Instructions:

1. Prepare Lemon-Garlic Marinade:

- Whisk together olive oil, fresh lemon juice, minced garlic, lemon zest, honey or maple syrup, dried oregano, salt, and pepper in a bowl. Set aside.

1. Marinate Shrimp:

- Place the peeled and deveined shrimp in a shallow dish and pour half of the Lemon-Garlic marinade over them. Toss to coat the shrimp evenly. Let them marinate in the refrigerator for at least 15-30 minutes.

1. Prepare Vegetables:

- While the shrimp is marinating, cut the bell peppers and zucchini into chunks or slices, depending on your preference.

1. Assemble Skewers:

- Thread marinated shrimp, bell pepper chunks, zucchini

slices, and cherry tomatoes onto the skewers in an alternating pattern.

1. Grill or Broil:

• Preheat the grill or broiler.

• Place the skewers on the grill or under the broiler, cooking for about 3-4 minutes per side or until the shrimp are opaque and the vegetables are slightly charred.

1. Baste with Marinade:

• Baste the skewers with the remaining Lemon-Garlic marinade for added flavor during grilling.

1. Serve:

• Once cooked, transfer the skewers to a serving platter.

• Drizzle with any remaining marinade and serve hot.

1. Enjoy your Shrimp and Vegetable Skewers with Lemon-Garlic Marinade!

Nutrition Information (per serving):

• Calories: 200

• Protein: 18g

• Fat: 12g

• Carbohydrates: 10g

• Fiber: 2g

• Sugar: 6g

• Sodium: 300mg

CHAPTER THREE

High-Calorie Recipes

Beef and Vegetable Stir-Fry with Brown Rice

Meal Description: Indulge in the rich flavors of this Beef and Vegetable Stir-Fry with Brown Rice, a hearty and wholesome meal that's quick and easy to prepare. Tender strips of beef are stir-fried with a colorful array of vegetables and tossed in a savory sauce, served alongside nutty brown rice for a satisfying and nutritious dish. Packed with protein, fiber, and essential nutrients, this stir-fry is perfect for a delicious weeknight dinner that the whole family will love.

Ingredients:

For Stir-Fry Sauce:

• 1/4 cup low-sodium soy sauce

• 2 tbsp oyster sauce

• 1 tbsp honey or maple syrup

• 1 tbsp rice vinegar

• 1 tsp sesame oil

• Two cloves garlic, minced

• 1 tsp grated ginger

• 1 tbsp cornstarch

• 1/4 cup water

For Beef and Vegetable Stir-Fry:

• 1 lb beef sirloin or flank steak, thinly sliced against the grain

• 2 tbsp vegetable oil, divided

• 2 cups mixed vegetables (such as bell peppers, broccoli,

carrots, snap peas)

• Cooked brown rice for serving

• Optional garnish: sliced green onions, sesame seeds

Instructions:

1. Prepare Stir-Fry Sauce:

• In a small bowl, whisk together low-sodium soy sauce, oyster sauce, honey or maple syrup, rice vinegar, sesame oil, minced garlic, grated ginger, cornstarch, and water until well combined. Set aside.

1. Prepare Beef and Vegetables:

• Heat one tablespoon of vegetable oil in a large skillet or wok over medium-high heat.

• Add thinly sliced beef to the skillet in a single layer and cook for 2-3 minutes per side or until browned and cooked to your desired doneness. Remove the meat from the skillet and set aside.

• In the same skillet, add another tablespoon of vegetable oil.

• Add mixed vegetables (such as bell peppers, broccoli, carrots, and snap peas) to the skillet and stir-fry for 4-5 minutes or until crisp-tender.

1. Combine and Cook:

• Return the cooked beef to the skillet with the vegetables.

• Pour the prepared stir-fry sauce over the beef and vegetables in the skillet.

• Cook for an additional 2-3 minutes or until the sauce has thickened and everything is heated through.

1. Serve:

• Serve the Beef and Vegetable Stir-Fry over cooked brown rice.

• Garnish with sliced green onions and sesame seeds if desired.

1. Enjoy your Beef and Vegetable Stir-Fry with Brown Rice!

Nutrition Information (per serving):

• Calories: 400

• Protein: 25g

• Fat: 15g

• Carbohydrates: 40g

• Fiber: 5g

• Sugar: 8g

• Sodium: 600mg

SALMON FILLET WITH ROASTED SWEET POTATOES AND ASPARAGUS

Meal Description: Treat yourself to a delectable and nutritious dinner with this Salmon Fillet with Roasted Sweet Potatoes and Asparagus. Fresh salmon fillets are seasoned and baked to perfection, while sweet potatoes and asparagus are roasted until tender and caramelized. This well-balanced meal is bursting with flavor and loaded with omega-3 fatty acids, vitamins, and minerals, making it a wholesome and satisfying option for any occasion.

Ingredients:

For Salmon:

• Four salmon fillets (6 oz each)

• 2 tbsp olive oil

• Two cloves garlic, minced

• 1 tsp dried thyme

• Salt and pepper to taste

• Lemon wedges for serving

For Roasted Sweet Potatoes:

• Two large sweet potatoes, peeled and diced

• 2 tbsp olive oil

• 1 tsp paprika

• 1/2 tsp garlic powder

• Salt and pepper to taste

For Roasted Asparagus:

• One bunch of asparagus, trimmed

• 2 tbsp olive oil

• Salt and pepper to taste

Instructions:

1. Preheat Oven:

• Preheat the oven to 400°F (200°C).

1. Prepare Salmon:

• Place the salmon fillets on a baking sheet lined with parchment paper.

• Mix olive oil, minced garlic, dried thyme, salt, and pepper in a small bowl.

• Brush the seasoned olive oil mixture over the salmon fillets.

• Squeeze fresh lemon juice over the salmon fillets.

1. Prepare Sweet Potatoes:

• Toss diced sweet potatoes with olive oil, paprika, garlic powder, salt, and pepper in a separate bowl until evenly coated.

• Spread the seasoned sweet potatoes in a single layer on another baking sheet lined with parchment paper.

1. Prepare Asparagus:

• Place trimmed asparagus on the same baking sheet as the sweet potatoes.

• Drizzle with olive oil, season with salt and pepper, and toss to coat.

1. Roast Everything:

• Transfer both baking sheets to the preheated oven.

• Roast the salmon fillets for 12-15 minutes or until cooked through and flaky.

• Roast the sweet potatoes and asparagus for 20-25 minutes, stirring halfway through, until tender and caramelized.

1. Serve:

• Once cooked, remove the salmon, sweet potatoes, and asparagus from the oven.

• Divide the salmon fillets, roasted sweet potatoes, and asparagus among serving plates.

• Serve hot, garnished with lemon wedges.

1. Enjoy your Salmon Fillet with Roasted Sweet Potatoes and Asparagus!

Nutrition Information (per serving):

• Calories: 400

• Protein: 30g

• Fat: 20g

• Carbohydrates: 25g

- Fiber: 6g
- Sugar: 7g
- Sodium: 300mg

CHICKEN ALFREDO PASTA WITH WHOLE WHEAT LINGUINE

Meal Description: Indulge in the creamy and comforting flavors of Chicken Alfredo Pasta with Whole Wheat Linguine. This wholesome version of the classic Alfredo dish features succulent chicken breast, whole wheat linguine, and a rich Alfredo sauce made with a blend of Parmesan cheese, garlic, and butter. Enjoy a satisfying and delicious meal that combines the indulgence of Alfredo with the nutritional benefits of whole wheat pasta and lean protein.

Ingredients:

For Chicken Alfredo:

• 8 oz whole wheat linguine

• Two boneless, skinless chicken breasts, thinly sliced

• 2 tbsp olive oil

• Three cloves garlic, minced

• 1 cup heavy cream

- 1 cup grated Parmesan cheese

- 4 tbsp unsalted butter

- Salt and pepper to taste

- Fresh parsley, chopped, for garnish (optional)

Instructions:

1. Cook Whole Wheat Linguine:

- Cook the whole wheat linguine according to the package instructions until al dente. Drain and set aside.

1. Cook Chicken:

- In a large skillet, heat olive oil over medium-high heat.

- Season thinly sliced chicken breasts with salt and pepper.

- Add the seasoned chicken to the skillet and cook until browned and cooked through, about 4-5 minutes per side.

- Remove the cooked chicken from the skillet and set aside.

1. Prepare Alfredo Sauce:

- In the same skillet, add minced garlic and cook for 1-2 minutes until fragrant.

- Reduce heat to medium-low and add butter to the skillet, allowing it to melt.

- Pour in the heavy cream and grated Parmesan cheese, stirring constantly until the cheese is melted and the sauce is smooth.

- Season with salt and pepper to taste.

1. Combine and Serve:

• Add the cooked whole wheat linguine to the Alfredo sauce, tossing to coat the pasta evenly.

• Slice the cooked chicken and arrange it over the Alfredo-coated linguine.

• Garnish with chopped fresh parsley if desired.

1. Serve your Chicken Alfredo Pasta with Whole Wheat Linguine hot and enjoy!

Nutrition Information (per serving):

• Calories: 550

• Protein: 30g

• Fat: 35g

• Carbohydrates: 35g

• Fiber: 6g

• Sugar: 2g

• Sodium: 400mg

QUINOA SALAD WITH AVOCADO, BLACK BEANS, AND CORN

Meal Description: Savor this Quinoa Salad's vibrant flavors and nutritious ingredients with Avocado, Black Beans, and Corn. Packed with protein, fiber, and healthy fats, this salad is not only delicious but also satisfying and wholesome. Nutty quinoa is combined with creamy avocado, hearty black beans, sweet corn, and a zesty lime-cilantro dressing, creating a refreshing and flavorful dish that's perfect for lunch or as a side for dinner.

Ingredients:

For Quinoa Salad:

- 1 cup quinoa, rinsed

- 2 cups water or vegetable broth

- One avocado, diced

- 1 cup cooked black beans (canned, rinsed and drained)

- 1 cup corn kernels (fresh or frozen, thawed)

- 1/4 cup red onion, finely chopped

- 1/4 cup fresh cilantro, chopped

- Salt and pepper to taste

For Lime-Cilantro Dressing:

- 3 tbsp olive oil

- 2 tbsp fresh lime juice

- One clove of garlic, minced

- 1 tsp honey or maple syrup

- 1/4 cup fresh cilantro, chopped

- Salt and pepper to taste

Instructions:

1. Cook Quinoa:

- In a saucepan, combine rinsed quinoa and water or vegetable broth.

- Bring to a boil, then reduce heat to low, cover, and simmer for 15-20 minutes until quinoa is tender and water is absorbed.

- Remove from heat and let the quinoa cool slightly.

1. Prepare Dressing:

- In a small bowl, whisk together olive oil, fresh lime juice, minced garlic, honey or maple syrup, chopped cilantro, salt, and pepper to make the dressing. Set aside.

1. Assemble Salad:

- In a large mixing bowl, combine cooked quinoa, diced avocado, black beans, corn kernels, finely chopped red onion, and chopped fresh cilantro.

- Pour the prepared lime-cilantro dressing over the salad ingredients.

- Gently toss to coat everything evenly in the dressing.

- Season with additional salt and pepper to taste if needed.

1. Chill and Serve:

- Cover the bowl and refrigerate the quinoa salad for at least 30 minutes to allow the flavors to meld together.

- Before serving, give the salad a final toss.

1. Enjoy your Quinoa Salad with Avocado, Black Beans, and Corn!

Nutrition Information (per serving):

- Calories: 350

- Protein: 10g

- Fat: 15g

- Carbohydrates: 45g

- Fiber: 10g

- Sugar: 4g

- Sodium: 300mg

BEEF AND BEAN CHILI WITH CHEESE AND SOUR CREAM

Meal Description: Warm up with a comforting bowl of Beef and Bean Chili topped with gooey cheese and creamy sour cream. This hearty chili is loaded with tender chunks of beef, kidney beans, tomatoes, and aromatic spices, creating a flavorful and satisfying meal that's perfect for chilly days. Topped with melted cheese and a dollop of sour cream, this classic dish is sure to please the whole family.

Ingredients:

For Beef and Bean Chili:

- 1 lb ground beef

- One onion, diced

- Three cloves garlic, minced

- One bell pepper, diced

- One can (14 oz) diced tomatoes

- One can (14 oz) kidney beans, drained and rinsed

- 1 cup beef broth

- 2 tbsp tomato paste

- 2 tsp chili powder
- 1 tsp cumin
- 1/2 tsp paprika
- Salt and pepper to taste

For Serving:

- Shredded cheddar cheese
- Sour cream
- Chopped green onions (optional)
- Tortilla chips or crusty bread (optional)

Instructions:

1. Brown Ground Beef:

- In a large pot or Dutch oven, brown the ground beef over medium heat, breaking it up with a spoon as it cooks.
- Once the beef is browned, remove any excess fat from the pot.

1. Cook Aromatics:

- Add diced onion, minced garlic, and diced bell pepper to the pot with the browned beef.
- Cook, stirring occasionally, until the vegetables are softened and fragrant.

1. Add Remaining Ingredients:

- Stir in diced tomatoes, kidney beans, beef broth, tomato paste, chili powder, cumin, paprika, salt, and pepper.
- Bring the chili to a simmer, then reduce heat to low and cook, uncovered, for about 30 minutes to allow the flavors to meld and the chili to thicken, stirring occasionally.

1. Serve:

• Ladle the hot chili into bowls.

• If desired, top each serving with shredded cheddar cheese, a dollop of sour cream, and chopped green onions.

• Serve with tortilla chips or crusty bread on the side for dipping.

1. Enjoy your Beef and Bean Chili with Cheese and Sour Cream!

Note: Feel free to customize the chili with your favorite toppings, such as avocado slices, jalapenos, or cilantro. Adjust the spice level by adding more or less chili powder and cumin according to your taste preferences.

CHICKEN AND VEGETABLE FAJITAS WITH GUACAMOLE AND TORTILLAS

Meal Description: Indulge in the sizzling flavors of Chicken and Vegetable Fajitas with Guacamole and Tortillas, a delicious and satisfying meal perfect for a weeknight dinner or casual gathering. Tender strips of seasoned chicken breast sautéed with bell peppers and onions are served with homemade guacamole and warm tortillas, creating a Tex-Mex feast that's bursting with flavor. Enjoy assembling your own fajitas with your favorite toppings for a customizable and enjoyable dining experience.

Ingredients:

For Chicken and Vegetables:

• 1 lb boneless, skinless chicken breast, thinly sliced

• Two bell peppers (any color), thinly sliced

• One onion, thinly sliced

- 2 tbsp olive oil

- Two cloves garlic, minced

- 1 tsp chili powder

- 1/2 tsp cumin

- 1/2 tsp paprika

- Salt and pepper to taste

For Guacamole:

- Two ripe avocados

- 1/4 cup diced tomato

- 2 tbsp finely chopped onion

- One clove of garlic, minced

- 1 tbsp lime juice

- 2 tbsp chopped fresh cilantro

- Salt and pepper to taste

For Serving:

- Eight small whole wheat or corn tortillas

- Optional toppings: shredded lettuce, diced tomatoes, shredded cheese, sour cream, salsa

Instructions:

1. Prepare Chicken and Vegetables:

- Heat olive oil over medium-high heat in a large skillet or grill pan.

- Add thinly sliced chicken breast to the skillet and season with minced garlic, chili powder, cumin, paprika, salt, and pepper. Cook until chicken is cooked through and browned about 5-6 minutes.

• Remove cooked chicken from the skillet and set aside.

• In the same skillet, add sliced bell peppers and onions. Sauté until tender-crisp, about 4-5 minutes. Remove from heat and set aside.

1. Make Guacamole:

• Mash the ripe avocados with a fork until smooth in a medium bowl.

• Add diced tomato, finely chopped onion, minced garlic, lime juice, chopped fresh cilantro, salt, and pepper. Stir until well combined.

1. Warm Tortillas:

• Heat the tortillas according to package instructions until warm and pliable. Keep warm until ready to serve.

1. Assemble Fajitas:

• Spread a spoonful of guacamole onto each warm tortilla.

• Top with a portion of cooked chicken and sautéed bell peppers and onions.

• You can add optional toppings such as shredded lettuce, diced tomatoes, shredded cheese, sour cream, and salsa as desired.

1. Roll up the tortillas and enjoy your Chicken and Vegetable Fajitas with Guacamole!

Nutrition Information (per serving - 2 fajitas):

• Calories: 230

• Protein: 20g

• Fat: 10g

• Carbohydrates: 15g

- Fiber: 5g
- Sugar: 2g
- Sodium: 200mg

SPAGHETTI CARBONARA WITH BACON, EGGS, AND PARMESAN CHEESE

Meal Description: Indulge in the rich and creamy flavors of Spaghetti Carbonara with Bacon, Eggs, and Parmesan Cheese, a classic Italian pasta dish that's both comforting and satisfying. Al dente spaghetti is tossed with crispy bacon, a creamy egg, Parmesan cheese sauce, and freshly cracked black pepper, creating a decadent and irresistible meal perfect for any occasion. Enjoy the simplicity and elegance of this timeless pasta dish that will indeed become a favorite in your repertoire.

Ingredients:

• 8 oz spaghetti

• Six slices bacon diced

• Three large eggs

• 3/4 cup grated Parmesan cheese, plus extra for serving

• Two cloves garlic, minced

• Freshly ground black pepper

• Chopped fresh parsley for garnish (optional)

Instructions:

1. Cook Spaghetti:

• Cook the spaghetti according to the package instructions until al dente. Drain, reserving 1/2 cup of pasta water, and set aside.

1. Cook Bacon:

• In a large skillet, cook the diced bacon over medium heat until crispy. Remove bacon from the skillet and place it on a plate lined with paper towels to drain excess grease. Reserve one tablespoon of bacon grease in the skillet.

1. Prepare Sauce:

• In a mixing bowl, whisk together the eggs, grated Parmesan cheese, minced garlic, and a generous amount of freshly ground black pepper.

1. Combine Everything:

• While the spaghetti is still hot, add it to the skillet with the reserved bacon grease. Toss to coat the spaghetti in the bacon grease.

• Quickly pour the egg and cheese mixture over the hot spaghetti, stirring continuously to coat the pasta evenly. The heat from the spaghetti will cook the eggs and create a creamy sauce. If the sauce is too thick, add some of the reserved pasta water to loosen it up.

• Add the cooked bacon to the skillet and toss to combine.

1. Serve:

• Transfer the spaghetti carbonara to serving plates.

• Garnish with additional grated Parmesan cheese,

freshly ground black pepper, and chopped fresh parsley if desired.

1. Enjoy your Spaghetti Carbonara with Bacon, Eggs, and Parmesan Cheese!

Nutrition Information (per serving):

- Calories: 450

- Protein: 22g

- Fat: 20g

- Carbohydrates: 40g

- Fiber: 2g

- Sugar: 2g

- Sodium: 600mg

STUFFED BELL PEPPERS WITH GROUND TURKEY, RICE, AND CHEESE

Meal Description: Delight your taste buds with these hearty and flavorful Stuffed Bell Peppers filled with a delicious mixture of ground turkey, rice, and cheese. These vibrant bell peppers are stuffed with a savory filling, baked to perfection, and topped with melted cheese, creating a satisfying and nutritious meal that's perfect for dinner. Packed with protein, fiber, and essential nutrients, these stuffed peppers are sure to become a family favorite.

Ingredients:

• Four large bell peppers (any color), tops removed and seeds removed

• 1 lb lean ground turkey

• 1 cup cooked rice (white or brown)

• 1/2 onion, diced

• Two cloves garlic, minced

• 1 cup tomato sauce

- 1 tsp dried oregano
- 1 tsp dried basil
- Salt and pepper to taste
- 1 cup shredded mozzarella cheese
- Chopped fresh parsley for garnish (optional)

Instructions:

1. Preheat Oven:

- Preheat the oven to 375°F (190°C). Lightly grease a baking dish large enough to hold the stuffed bell peppers.

1. Prepare Bell Peppers:

- Cut the tops off the bell peppers and remove the seeds and membranes from the inside. Rinse the peppers under cold water and set them aside.

1. Prepare Filling:

- In a large skillet, cook the ground turkey over medium heat until browned and cooked through, breaking it up with a spoon as it cooks.

- Add diced onion and minced garlic to the skillet with the cooked turkey. Cook for 2-3 minutes until the onion is translucent and fragrant.

- Stir in the cooked rice, tomato sauce, dried oregano, dried basil, salt, and pepper. Cook for an additional 2-3 minutes, allowing the flavors to blend.

1. Stuff Peppers:

- Spoon the turkey and rice mixture evenly into each hollowed-out bell pepper, pressing down gently to pack the filling.

- Place the stuffed bell peppers upright in the prepared

baking dish.

1. Bake:

• Cover the baking dish with aluminum foil and bake in the preheated oven for 25-30 minutes or until the bell peppers are tender.

1. Add Cheese:

• Remove the foil from the baking dish and sprinkle shredded mozzarella cheese evenly over the tops of the stuffed bell peppers.

• Return the baking dish to the oven and bake, uncovered, for an additional 5-7 minutes or until the cheese is melted and bubbly.

1. Serve:

• Remove the stuffed bell peppers from the oven and let them cool slightly.

• Garnish with chopped fresh parsley if desired.

• Serve hot, and enjoy your Stuffed Bell Peppers with Ground Turkey, Rice, and Cheese!

Nutrition Information (per serving - 1 stuffed bell pepper):

• Calories: 300

• Protein: 25g

• Fat: 10g

• Carbohydrates: 25g

• Fiber: 4g

• Sugar: 6g

• Sodium: 400mg

CHAPTER FOUR

Low-Carb Recipes

Cauliflower Crust Pizza with Tomato Sauce, Mozzarella, and Vegetables

Meal Description: Indulge in a healthier twist on a classic favorite with this Cauliflower Crust Pizza topped with rich tomato sauce, gooey mozzarella cheese, and an array of colorful vegetables. The cauliflower crust provides a nutritious and gluten-free base, while the savory toppings add flavor and freshness to every bite. Enjoy a guilt-free pizza night with this delicious and satisfying meal that's perfect for sharing with family and friends.

Ingredients:

For Cauliflower Crust:

• One medium head cauliflower, riced (about 4 cups)

• One egg, beaten

• 1/2 cup shredded mozzarella cheese

• 1/4 cup grated Parmesan cheese

• 1 tsp dried oregano

• 1/2 tsp garlic powder

• Salt and pepper to taste

For Pizza Toppings:

• 1/2 cup tomato sauce or pizza sauce

• 1 cup shredded mozzarella cheese

• Assorted vegetables (such as bell peppers, mushrooms, onions, olives, cherry tomatoes), sliced

• Fresh basil leaves for garnish (optional)

Instructions:

1. Preheat Oven:

• Preheat the oven to 425°F (220°C). Line a baking sheet or pizza pan with parchment paper.

1. Prepare Cauliflower Crust:

• Place the riced cauliflower in a microwave-safe bowl and microwave on high for 5-6 minutes until tender. Allow the cauliflower to cool slightly.

• Transfer the cooked cauliflower to a clean kitchen towel or cheesecloth and squeeze out as much moisture as possible.

• Combine the squeezed cauliflower in a large mixing bowl with beaten egg, shredded mozzarella cheese, grated Parmesan cheese, dried oregano, garlic powder, salt, and pepper. Mix until well combined.

• Press the cauliflower mixture evenly onto the prepared baking sheet or pizza pan, forming a crust about 1/4 inch thick.

1. Bake Crust:

• Bake the cauliflower crust in the preheated oven for 20-25 minutes or until it is golden brown and firm to the touch.

1. Add Toppings:

• Remove the cauliflower crust from the oven and spread tomato sauce evenly over the crust, leaving a small border around the edges.

• Sprinkle shredded mozzarella cheese over the tomato sauce.

• Arrange sliced vegetables over the cheese.

1. Bake Pizza:

• Return the pizza to the oven and bake for an additional 10-15 minutes, or until the cheese is melted and bubbly and the crust is crispy.

1. Serve:

• Remove the cauliflower crust pizza from the oven and let it cool slightly.

• Garnish with fresh basil leaves if desired.

• Slice and serve hot.

Nutrition Information (per serving - 1/4 of the pizza):

• Calories: 200

• Protein: 12g

• Fat: 10g

• Carbohydrates: 15g

• Fiber: 5g

• Sugar: 5g

• Sodium: 400mg

EGGPLANT LASAGNA WITH RICOTTA, SPINACH, AND MARINARA SAUCE

Meal Description: Savor the rich and comforting flavors of this Eggplant Lasagna, which features layers of tender eggplant, creamy ricotta cheese, spinach, and marinara sauce. This lighter twist on traditional lasagna swaps out the pasta for thinly sliced eggplant, making it a low-carb and gluten-free option that's still hearty and satisfying. Whether you're looking for a meatless meal or want to incorporate more vegetables into your diet, this eggplant lasagna is sure to become a new favorite.

Ingredients:

- Two large eggplants, thinly sliced lengthwise

- 2 cups marinara sauce (homemade or store-bought)

- 1 cup part-skim ricotta cheese

- 1 cup shredded mozzarella cheese

- 1 cup chopped spinach

- 1/4 cup grated Parmesan cheese

- Two cloves garlic, minced

- 1 tsp dried oregano

- 1/2 tsp dried basil

- Salt and pepper to taste

- Olive oil for greasing

Instructions:

1. Preheat Oven:

- Preheat the oven to 375°F (190°C). Grease a 9x13-inch baking dish with olive oil.

1. Prepare Eggplant:

- Slice the eggplants lengthwise into thin slices, about 1/4 inch thick.

- Place the eggplant slices on a baking sheet lined with parchment paper. Sprinkle both sides with salt and let them sit for about 10 minutes to release excess moisture.

- After 10 minutes, blot the eggplant slices with paper towels to remove the excess moisture.

1. Assemble Layers:

- Spread a thin layer of marinara sauce on the bottom of the prepared baking dish.

- Arrange a layer of eggplant slices over the marinara sauce.

- Combine ricotta cheese, chopped spinach, minced garlic, dried oregano, dried basil, salt, and pepper in a mixing bowl. Mix until well combined.

- Spread half of the ricotta and spinach mixture over the

eggplant layer.

• Sprinkle a layer of shredded mozzarella cheese over the ricotta mixture.

• Repeat the layers: marinara sauce, eggplant slices, remaining ricotta and spinach mixture, and shredded mozzarella cheese.

1. Bake:

• Cover the baking dish with aluminum foil and bake in the preheated oven for 30 minutes.

• After 30 minutes, remove the foil and sprinkle grated Parmesan cheese over the top of the lasagna.

• Return the lasagna to the oven and bake, uncovered for 15-20 minutes, or until the cheese is melted and bubbly and the eggplant is tender.

1. Serve:

• Remove the eggplant lasagna from the oven and let it cool slightly before slicing.

• Garnish with fresh basil leaves if desired.

• Serve hot and enjoy!

Nutrition Information (per serving):

• Calories: 250

• Protein: 15g

• Fat: 12g

• Carbohydrates: 20g

• Fiber: 8g

• Sugar: 10g

• Sodium: 600mg

ZUCCHINI BOATS STUFFED WITH GROUND TURKEY AND CHEESE

Meal Description: Experience a delicious and nutritious twist on classic stuffed peppers with these Zucchini Boats filled with seasoned ground turkey and melted cheese. Zucchini halves serve as the perfect vessel for a flavorful mixture of lean ground turkey, aromatic spices, and gooey melted cheese. This low-carb and protein-packed dish is sure to satisfy your cravings while providing a healthy alternative to traditional stuffed peppers. Enjoy these zucchini boats as a wholesome meal that's easy to prepare and bursting with flavor.

Ingredients:

- Four medium zucchinis

- 1 lb lean ground turkey

- 1/2 onion, diced

- Two cloves garlic, minced

- One bell pepper, diced

- 1 cup marinara sauce

- 1 cup shredded mozzarella cheese

- 2 tbsp olive oil

- 1 tsp dried oregano

- 1/2 tsp dried basil

- Salt and pepper to taste

- Fresh parsley for garnish (optional)

Instructions:

1. Preheat Oven:

- Preheat the oven to 375°F (190°C). Grease a baking dish large enough to hold the zucchini boats.

1. Prepare Zucchini Boats:

- Cut each zucchini in half lengthwise. Use a spoon to scoop out the seeds and create a hollowed-out "boat" shape. Place the hollowed zucchini halves in the prepared baking dish.

1. Prepare Filling:

- Heat olive oil in a large skillet over medium heat. Add diced onion and minced garlic, and cook until softened and fragrant.

- Add ground turkey to the skillet and cook until browned, breaking it up with a spoon as it cooks.

- Stir in diced bell pepper, dried oregano, dried basil, salt, and pepper. Cook for an additional 2-3 minutes.

- Pour marinara sauce over the turkey mixture and stir until well combined. Simmer for 5 minutes.

1. Assemble Zucchini Boats:

- Spoon the turkey and marinara mixture evenly into the

hollowed-out zucchini halves, pressing down gently to pack the filling.

• Sprinkle shredded mozzarella cheese over the top of each zucchini boat.

1. Bake:

• Cover the baking dish with aluminum foil and bake in the preheated oven for 20-25 minutes, or until the zucchini is tender and the cheese is melted and bubbly.

1. Serve:

• Remove the zucchini boats from the oven and let them cool slightly.

• Garnish with fresh parsley if desired.

• Serve hot and enjoy your Zucchini Boats Stuffed with Ground Turkey and Cheese!

Nutrition Information (per serving - 1 zucchini boat):

• Calories: 250

• Protein: 20g

• Fat: 10g

• Carbohydrates: 15g

• Fiber: 5g

• Sugar: 8g

• Sodium: 400mg

BAKED CHICKEN THIGHS WITH BRUSSELS SPROUTS AND BACON

Meal Description: Delight your taste buds with this flavorful and satisfying dish of Baked Chicken Thighs with Brussels Sprouts and Bacon. Succulent chicken thighs are seasoned to perfection, accompanied by tender roasted Brussels sprouts and crispy bacon, creating a hearty and wholesome meal that's easy to prepare and full of comforting flavors. Whether you're looking for a simple weeknight dinner or a comforting meal to share with loved ones, this dish is sure to impress.

Ingredients:

For Baked Chicken Thighs:

• Four bone-in, skin-on chicken thighs

• 2 tbsp olive oil

• Two cloves garlic, minced

• 1 tsp dried thyme

- 1 tsp dried rosemary

- Salt and pepper to taste

For Brussels Sprouts and Bacon:

- 1 lb Brussels sprouts, trimmed and halved

- Four slices of bacon diced

- 2 tbsp balsamic vinegar

- Salt and pepper to taste

Instructions:

1. Preheat Oven:

- Preheat the oven to 400°F (200°C). Grease a baking dish large enough to hold the chicken thighs and Brussels sprouts.

1. Prepare Chicken Thighs:

- In a small bowl, combine olive oil, minced garlic, dried thyme, dried rosemary, salt, and pepper to create a marinade.

- Place the chicken thighs in the prepared baking dish. Brush the marinade over the chicken thighs, coating them evenly.

1. Prepare Brussels Sprouts and Bacon:

- Toss halved Brussels sprouts with diced bacon and balsamic vinegar in a separate bowl until well combined. Season with salt and pepper to taste.

- Arrange the Brussels sprouts and bacon mixture around the chicken thighs in the baking dish.

1. Bake:

- Transfer the baking dish to the preheated oven and bake

for 35-40 minutes, or until the chicken thighs are golden brown and cooked through and the Brussels sprouts are tender, stirring the Brussels sprouts halfway through cooking.

1. Serve:

• Remove the baked chicken thighs and Brussels sprouts from the oven.

• Transfer the chicken thighs to a serving platter and spoon the Brussels sprouts and bacon mixture alongside.

• Serve hot, and enjoy your Baked Chicken Thighs with Brussels Sprouts and Bacon!

Nutrition Information (per serving - 1 chicken thigh with Brussels sprouts and bacon):

• Calories: 350

• Protein: 25g

• Fat: 20g

• Carbohydrates: 15g

• Fiber: 5g

• Sugar: 3g

• Sodium: 400mg

BROCCOLI AND CHEDDAR SOUP WITH CHICKEN

Meal Description: Warm up on chilly days with a comforting bowl of broccoli and cheddar soup with chicken. This hearty and delicious meal is sure to satisfy your cravings. Tender pieces of chicken, fresh broccoli florets, and creamy cheddar cheese come together in a flavorful broth, creating a nutritious and indulgent soup. Whether enjoyed as a comforting lunch or a cozy dinner, this soup is bound to become a favorite in your household.

Ingredients:

• 1 lb boneless, skinless chicken breasts, diced

• 4 cups broccoli florets

• One onion, diced

• Two cloves garlic, minced

• 4 cups chicken broth

• 1 cup milk (any kind)

• 1 cup shredded cheddar cheese

• 2 tbsp butter

• 2 tbsp all-purpose flour

• Salt and pepper to taste

• Chopped fresh parsley for garnish (optional)

Instructions:

1. Cook Chicken:

• In a large pot, heat olive oil over medium heat. Add diced chicken breasts and cook until browned and cooked through about 5-6 minutes. Remove the cooked chicken from the pot and set aside.

1. Sauté Vegetables:

• In the same pot, melt butter over medium heat. Add diced onion and minced garlic, and cook until softened and fragrant.

• Add broccoli florets to the pot and cook for an additional 3-4 minutes until slightly tender.

1. Make Roux:

• Sprinkle all-purpose flour over the vegetables in the pot and stir to combine, creating a roux.

• Cook the roux for 1-2 minutes, constantly stirring, until golden brown.

1. Add Broth and Simmer:

• Slowly pour chicken broth into the pot, stirring continuously to prevent lumps from forming.

• Bring the soup to a simmer and cook for 10-12 minutes, until the broccoli is tender.

1. Blend Soup:

• Blend the soup until smooth and creamy using an immersion blender. Alternatively, transfer the soup to a blender and blend in batches until smooth. Return the blended soup to the pot.

1. Add Chicken and Cheese:

• Return the cooked chicken to the pot with the blended soup.

• Stir in milk and shredded cheddar cheese until the cheese is melted and the soup is heated through.

• Season with salt and pepper to taste.

1. Serve:

• Ladle the Broccoli and Cheddar Soup with Chicken into serving bowls.

• Garnish with chopped fresh parsley if desired.

• Serve hot and enjoy!

Nutrition Information (per serving):

• Calories: 300

• Protein: 25g

• Fat: 15g

• Carbohydrates: 15g

• Fiber: 3g

• Sugar: 5g

• Sodium: 700mg

CABBAGE STIR-FRY WITH GROUND BEEF AND SOY SAUCE

Meal Description: Indulge in the savory goodness of this Cabbage Stir-Fry with Ground Beef and Soy Sauce —a quick, easy, and flavorful dish perfect for busy weeknights. Crispy cabbage, seasoned ground beef, and a delicious soy sauce glaze combine in a delightful medley of textures and tastes. Packed with protein and vegetables, this stir-fry is satisfying and a wholesome addition to your dinner repertoire.

Ingredients:

- 1 lb ground beef
- One small cabbage, thinly sliced
- One onion, thinly sliced
- Three cloves garlic, minced
- 2 tbsp vegetable oil
- 1/4 cup soy sauce
- 2 tbsp oyster sauce

- 1 tbsp sesame oil

- 1 tsp ginger, grated

- 1/2 tsp red pepper flakes (optional)

- Salt and pepper to taste

- Green onions, chopped, for garnish (optional)

- Sesame seeds for garnish (optional)

Instructions:

1. Cook Ground Beef:

- Heat vegetable oil in a large skillet or wok over medium-high heat. Add ground beef and cook until browned, breaking it up with a spoon as you go.

1. Add Aromatics:

- Add thinly sliced onions and minced garlic to the skillet with the cooked ground beef. Stir-fry for 2-3 minutes until the onions are softened and aromatic.

1. Stir-Fry Cabbage:

- Add the thinly sliced cabbage to the skillet. Stir-fry the cabbage and beef mixture for 5-7 minutes or until the cabbage is crisp-tender and slightly caramelized.

1. Prepare Soy Sauce Glaze:

- In a small bowl, whisk together soy sauce, oyster sauce, sesame oil, grated ginger, and red pepper flakes if using.

1. Combine and Season:

- Pour the soy sauce glaze over the cabbage and beef mixture. Toss everything together to coat evenly. Season with salt and pepper to taste.

1. Finish Cooking:

• Continue to stir-fry for an additional 2-3 minutes, allowing the flavors to meld and the cabbage to absorb the sauce.

1. Garnish and Serve:

• Garnish the Cabbage Stir-Fry with chopped green onions and sesame seeds if desired.

• Serve hot over rice or noodles.

Nutrition Information (per serving):

• Calories: 350

• Protein: 25g

• Fat: 22g

• Carbohydrates: 15g

• Fiber: 5g

• Sugar: 8g

• Sodium: 800mg

KETO CHICKEN TENDERS WITH ALMOND FLOUR BREADING

Meal Description: Indulge in crispy and flavorful Keto Chicken Tenders with Almond Flour Bread, a low-carb twist on a classic favorite perfect for those following a ketogenic lifestyle. These tender chicken strips are coated in a crunchy almond flour breading, seasoned to perfection, and baked to golden perfection. Enjoy them as a delicious appetizer, snack, or main dish paired with your favorite dipping sauce for a satisfying and guilt-free meal.

Ingredients:

• 1 lb boneless, skinless chicken breasts cut into strips

• 1 cup almond flour

• Two eggs

• 1 tsp garlic powder

• 1 tsp paprika

• 1/2 tsp onion powder

- 1/2 tsp dried oregano

- 1/2 tsp salt

- 1/4 tsp black pepper

- Cooking spray or olive oil for greasing

Instructions:

1. Preheat Oven:

- Preheat the oven to 400°F (200°C). Line a baking sheet with parchment paper and lightly grease with cooking spray or olive oil.

1. Prepare Breading Station:

- Whisk together the eggs in a shallow bowl or dish until well beaten.

- Combine almond flour, garlic powder, paprika, onion powder, dried oregano, salt, and black pepper in another shallow bowl or dish. Mix well.

1. Coat Chicken Strips:

- Dip each chicken strip into the beaten eggs, allowing any excess to drip off.

- Coat the chicken strip in the almond flour mixture, pressing gently to adhere the breading to the chicken. Ensure that the chicken strip is evenly coated on all sides.

1. Arrange on Baking Sheet:

- Place the breaded chicken strips on the prepared baking sheet in a single layer, leaving some space between each strip.

1. Bake:

- Bake the chicken tenders in the oven for 15-20 minutes or until the chicken is cooked and the breading is golden and crispy.

1. Serve:

• Remove the Keto Chicken Tenders from the oven and let them cool slightly.

• Serve hot with your favorite dipping sauce, such as sugar-free barbecue sauce, ranch dressing, or mustard.

Nutrition Information (per serving - 4 chicken tenders):

• Calories: 300

• Protein: 30g

• Fat: 15g

• Carbohydrates: 5g

• Fiber: 3g

• Sugar: 1g

• Sodium: 500mg

SPINACH AND MUSHROOM CRUSTLESS QUICHE

Meal Description: Delight in a flavorful and nutritious Spinach and Mushroom Crustless Quiche—a versatile dish that's perfect for breakfast, brunch, or even dinner. Packed with sautéed mushrooms, tender spinach, and creamy cheese, this crustless quiche is both satisfying and wholesome. Enjoy it warm or at room temperature, whether served as a main dish or sliced into smaller portions for a delightful appetizer or side dish.

Ingredients:

• 1 tbsp olive oil

• One onion, diced

• Two cloves garlic, minced

• 8 oz mushrooms, sliced

• 4 cups fresh spinach leaves

• Six large eggs

• 1/2 cup milk (any kind)

• 1 cup shredded cheese (such as cheddar, mozzarella, or Swiss)

• 1/4 tsp dried thyme

• Salt and pepper to taste

Instructions:

1. Preheat Oven:

• Preheat the oven to 375°F (190°C). Grease a 9-inch pie dish or quiche pan with cooking spray or olive oil.

1. Sauté Vegetables:

• Heat olive oil in a large skillet over medium heat. Add diced onion and minced garlic, and cook until softened and fragrant.

• Add sliced mushrooms to the skillet and cook until they release their moisture and become tender, about 5-7 minutes.

• Add fresh spinach leaves to the skillet and cook until wilted, stirring occasionally. Remove the skillet from heat and set aside.

1. Prepare Egg Mixture:

• In a large mixing bowl, whisk together eggs, milk, dried thyme, salt, and pepper until well combined.

1. Assemble Quiche:

• Spread the sautéed mushroom and spinach mixture evenly on the bottom of the greased pie dish or quiche pan.

• Sprinkle shredded cheese over the mushroom and spinach mixture.

1. Pour Egg Mixture:

• Pour the egg mixture evenly over the vegetables and cheese in the pie dish or quiche pan.

1. Bake:

• Transfer the quiche to the preheated oven and bake for 25-30 minutes, or until the center is set and the top is golden brown.

1. Serve:

• Remove the Spinach and Mushroom Crustless Quiche from the oven and let it cool slightly before slicing.

• Serve warm or at room temperature, garnished with fresh herbs if desired.

Nutrition Information (per serving - 1/6 of the quiche):

• Calories: 180

• Protein: 12g

• Fat: 12g

• Carbohydrates: 6g

• Fiber: 2g

• Sugar: 2g

• Sodium: 300mg

CHAPTER FIVE

High-Carb Recipes

Spaghetti Squash Pad Thai with Shrimp and Peanuts

Meal Description: Experience the vibrant flavors of Thailand with this unique and flavorful Spaghetti Squash Pad Thai with Shrimp and Peanuts. This lighter twist on the classic dish is delicious and nutritious. Tender strands of spaghetti squash are tossed with succulent shrimp, crisp vegetables, and a tangy-sweet Pad Thai sauce, then garnished with crunchy peanuts and fresh cilantro. Enjoy this satisfying meal that's sure to become a favorite in your recipe collection.

Ingredients:

• One medium spaghetti squash

• 1 lb medium shrimp, peeled and deveined

• Two cloves garlic, minced

• 1 red bell pepper, julienned

• One carrot, julienned

• Two green onions, thinly sliced

• 1/4 cup chopped peanuts

• Fresh cilantro leaves for garnish

For Pad Thai Sauce:

• 3 tbsp soy sauce (or tamari for gluten-free)

• 2 tbsp fish sauce

• 2 tbsp rice vinegar

• 2 tbsp lime juice

• 2 tbsp brown sugar (or coconut sugar for low-carb)

• 1 tbsp sriracha sauce (adjust to taste)

• 1 tbsp sesame oil

Instructions:

1. Prepare Spaghetti Squash:

• Preheat the oven to 400°F (200°C). Cut the spaghetti squash in half lengthwise and scoop out the seeds with a spoon. Place the squash halves, cut side down, on a baking sheet lined with parchment paper. Bake for 30-40 minutes or until the squash is tender and the flesh can be easily shredded with a fork. Let cool slightly.

1. Shred Squash:

• Scrape the cooked spaghetti squash flesh into strands using a fork. Transfer the strands to a large bowl and set aside.

1. Make Pad Thai Sauce:

• In a small bowl, whisk together soy sauce, fish sauce, rice vinegar, lime juice, brown sugar, sriracha sauce, and sesame oil until well combined. Set aside.

1. Cook Shrimp:

• In a large skillet or wok, heat some oil over medium-high heat. Add minced garlic and cook until fragrant. Add shrimp and cook until pink and opaque, about 2-3 minutes per side. Remove the shrimp from the skillet and set aside.

1. Sauté Vegetables:

• In the same skillet, add julienned red bell pepper and carrot. Stir-fry for 2-3 minutes until slightly softened.

1. Assemble Pad Thai:

• Add the cooked spaghetti squash strands to the skillet with the sautéed vegetables. Pour the Pad Thai sauce over the squash and vegetables. Toss everything together until well coated and heated through.

1. Add Shrimp and Garnish:

• Return the cooked shrimp to the skillet with the squash and vegetables. Stir to combine.

• Sprinkle chopped peanuts and sliced green onions over the Pad Thai. Garnish with fresh cilantro leaves.

1. Serve:

• Divide the Spaghetti Squash Pad Thai with Shrimp and Peanuts among serving plates.

• Serve hot and enjoy!

Nutrition Information (per serving):

• Calories: 250

• Protein: 20g

• Fat: 10g

• Carbohydrates: 20g

• Fiber: 5g

• Sugar: 10g

• Sodium: 800mg

QUINOA AND BLACK BEAN BURRITO BOWL WITH SALSA AND GUACAMOLE

Meal Description: Indulge in a burst of Mexican-inspired flavors with this wholesome and satisfying Quinoa and Black Bean Burrito Bowl with Salsa and Guacamole—a vibrant and nutritious meal that's perfect for lunch or dinner. Protein-packed quinoa and black beans are combined with colorful vegetables, zesty salsa, creamy guacamole, and tangy lime for a burst of freshness in every bite. Customize your bowl with your favorite toppings and enjoy a delicious and filling meal that's sure to satisfy your cravings.

Ingredients:

• 1 cup quinoa, rinsed

• One can (15 oz) black beans, drained and rinsed

• One red bell pepper, diced

• 1 cup corn kernels (fresh or frozen)

- 1/2 red onion, finely chopped

- One jalapeño, seeded and minced

- 1/4 cup chopped fresh cilantro

- Juice of 1 lime

- Salt and pepper to taste

- Salsa, for serving

- Guacamole, for serving

- Optional toppings: diced tomatoes, shredded lettuce, sliced black olives, shredded cheese, Greek yogurt or sour cream

Instructions:

1. Cook Quinoa:

- In a medium saucepan, bring 2 cups of water to a boil. Add rinsed quinoa and a pinch of salt. Reduce heat to low, cover, and simmer for 15-20 minutes or until the quinoa is tender and the water is absorbed. Remove from heat and let it sit, covered, for 5 minutes. Fluff with a fork.

1. Prepare Black Bean Mixture:

- In a separate skillet, heat some oil over medium heat. Add diced red bell pepper, corn kernels, finely chopped red onion, and minced jalapeño. Sauté for 5-7 minutes or until the vegetables are softened.

- Add drained and rinsed black beans to the skillet with the vegetables. Cook for an additional 2-3 minutes to heat through.

1. Combine Quinoa and Black Bean Mixture:

- Transfer the cooked quinoa to a large mixing bowl. Add the black bean and vegetable mixture to the bowl.

• Add chopped fresh cilantro and squeeze the juice of one lime over the mixture. Season with salt and pepper to taste. Toss everything together until well combined.

1. Assemble Burrito Bowls:

• Divide the quinoa and black bean mixture evenly among serving bowls.

• Top each bowl with salsa and guacamole.

• You can add any desired optional toppings, such as diced tomatoes, shredded lettuce, sliced black olives, shredded cheese, Greek yogurt, or sour cream.

1. Serve:

• Serve the Quinoa and Black Bean Burrito Bowls immediately.

• Enjoy hot or refrigerated leftovers for a delicious cold lunch the next day.

Nutrition Information (per serving):

• Calories: 350

• Protein: 15g

• Fat: 10g

• Carbohydrates: 50g

• Fiber: 10g

• Sugar: 5g

• Sodium: 500mg

SWEET POTATO AND BLACK BEAN ENCHILADAS WITH RED SAUCE

Meal Description: Savor the bold and comforting flavors of Mexican cuisine with these Sweet Potato and Black Bean Enchiladas with Red Sauce. This delightful vegetarian dish is hearty, nutritious, and bursting with flavor. Soft tortillas are filled with a savory mixture of roasted sweet potatoes, protein-rich black beans, and melted cheese, then smothered in a tangy, aromatic red enchilada sauce. Serve these enchiladas with your favorite toppings for a satisfying meal that's sure to please everyone at the dinner table.

Ingredients:

• Two medium sweet potatoes, peeled and diced

• One can (15 oz) black beans, drained and rinsed

• 1 onion, diced

• Two cloves garlic, minced

• 1 tsp ground cumin

• 1 tsp chili powder

- 1/2 tsp smoked paprika

- Salt and pepper to taste

- Eight small flour tortillas

- 2 cups red enchilada sauce

- 1 1/2 cups shredded cheese (such as cheddar or Monterey Jack)

- Fresh cilantro, chopped, for garnish

- Sour cream or Greek yogurt for serving (optional)

- Sliced avocado for serving (optional)

Instructions:

1. Roast Sweet Potatoes:

- Preheat the oven to 400°F (200°C). Place diced sweet potatoes on a baking sheet lined with parchment paper. Drizzle with olive oil and sprinkle with salt and pepper. Roast in the preheated oven for 20-25 minutes or until tender and lightly browned.

1. Prepare Filling:

- Heat oil in a large skillet over medium heat. Add diced onion and minced garlic, and cook until softened and fragrant.

- Add drained and rinsed black beans, ground cumin, chili powder, smoked paprika, salt, and pepper to the skillet and stir to combine.

- Add the roasted sweet potatoes to the skillet and gently mash some of them with a fork. Stir to combine all ingredients. Remove from heat and set aside.

1. Assemble Enchiladas:

- Spread a small amount of red enchilada sauce on the

bottom of a baking dish.

• Place a spoonful of the sweet potato and black bean mixture onto each flour tortilla. Sprinkle some shredded cheese over the filling.

• Roll up the tortillas and place them seam-side down in the prepared baking dish.

1. Top with Sauce and Cheese:

• Pour the remaining red enchilada sauce over the rolled tortillas in the baking dish, covering them evenly.

• Sprinkle the remaining shredded cheese over the top of the enchiladas.

1. Bake:

• Cover the baking dish with aluminum foil and bake in the preheated oven for 20-25 minutes, or until the enchiladas are heated through and the cheese is melted and bubbly.

1. Serve:

• Remove the Sweet Potato and Black Bean Enchiladas from the oven and let them cool slightly.

• Garnish with chopped fresh cilantro.

• Serve hot with optional toppings such as sour cream, Greek yogurt, and sliced avocado.

Nutrition Information (per serving - 2 enchiladas):

• Calories: 400

• Protein: 15g

• Fat: 15g

• Carbohydrates: 50g

- Fiber: 10g
- Sugar: 5g
- Sodium: 800mg

WHOLE WHEAT PASTA PRIMAVERA WITH VEGETABLES AND PESTO

Meal Description: Indulge in the vibrant flavors of spring with this wholesome and satisfying Whole Wheat Pasta Primavera with Vegetables and Pesto—a delightful dish that celebrates the season's bounty. Colorful vegetables, including bell peppers, cherry tomatoes, zucchini, and broccoli, are sautéed to perfection, tossed with whole wheat pasta, and coated in a flavorful homemade pesto sauce. Enjoy this nutritious and delicious meal that's perfect for lunch or dinner, whether served hot or cold.

Ingredients:

For Pesto Sauce:

• 2 cups fresh basil leaves

• 1/2 cup grated Parmesan cheese

• 1/4 cup pine nuts or walnuts

• Two cloves garlic, minced

• 1/2 cup extra virgin olive oil

- Salt and pepper to taste

For Pasta Primavera:

- 8 oz whole wheat pasta (such as penne or fusilli)
- One red bell pepper, thinly sliced
- One yellow bell pepper, thinly sliced
- One zucchini, thinly sliced
- 1 cup cherry tomatoes, halved
- 1 cup broccoli florets
- 2 tbsp olive oil
- Salt and pepper to taste
- Grated Parmesan cheese for serving (optional)

Instructions:

1. Prepare Pesto Sauce:

- Combine fresh basil leaves, grated Parmesan cheese, pine nuts or walnuts, minced garlic, salt, and pepper in a food processor or blender.

- With the food processor running, gradually drizzle in the extra virgin olive oil until the pesto is smooth and creamy. Taste and adjust the seasoning as needed. Set aside.

1. Cook Pasta:

- Cook the whole wheat pasta according to the package instructions until al dente. Drain and set aside, reserving some pasta cooking water.

1. Sauté Vegetables:

- Heat olive oil in a large skillet over medium heat. Add thinly sliced red and yellow bell peppers, zucchini, cherry tomatoes, and broccoli florets to the skillet. Sauté for 5-7 minutes or until the vegetables are tender-crisp. Season with salt and pepper to taste.

1. Combine Pasta and Vegetables:

• Add the cooked whole wheat pasta to the skillet with the sautéed vegetables. Toss everything together until well combined.

1. Add Pesto Sauce:

• Pour the prepared pesto sauce over the pasta and vegetables. Toss to coat evenly, adding some reserved pasta cooking water if needed to loosen the sauce and create a creamy consistency.

1. Serve:

• Transfer the Whole Wheat Pasta Primavera with Vegetables and Pesto to serving plates or bowls.

• Sprinkle with grated Parmesan cheese if desired.

• Serve hot or cold, as desired.

Nutrition Information (per serving):

• Calories: 400

• Protein: 12g

• Fat: 20g

• Carbohydrates: 45g

• Fiber: 8g

• Sugar: 5g

• Sodium: 300mg

LENTIL SOUP WITH CARROTS, CELERY, AND POTATOES

Meal Description: Warm up with a comforting bowl of Lentil Soup with Carrots, Celery, and Potatoes—a hearty and nutritious dish that's perfect for chilly days. This wholesome soup features protein-rich lentils simmered with aromatic vegetables, including carrots, celery, and potatoes, in a flavorful broth seasoned with herbs and spices. Whether enjoyed as a light lunch or a cozy dinner, this soup is sure to nourish your body and soul.

Ingredients:

• 1 cup dried green or brown lentils, rinsed and drained

• Two carrots diced

• 2 celery stalks, diced

• One onion, diced

• Two cloves garlic, minced

• 2 potatoes, diced

• 6 cups vegetable or chicken broth

• One bay leaf

• 1 tsp dried thyme

- 1 tsp dried oregano
- Salt and pepper to taste
- Olive oil for cooking
- Fresh parsley for garnish (optional)
- Lemon wedges for serving (optional)

Instructions:

1. Prepare Vegetables:

- Heat olive oil in a large pot over medium heat. Add diced onion, carrots, and celery. Sauté for 5-7 minutes or until the vegetables are softened.

1. Add Lentils and Spices:

- Add minced garlic, dried thyme, and dried oregano to the pot. Stir and cook for another minute, until fragrant.

1. Simmer Soup:

- Add rinsed and drained lentils, diced potatoes, bay leaf, and vegetable or chicken broth to the pot. Stir to combine.
- Bring the soup to a boil, then reduce the heat to low. Cover and simmer for 20-25 minutes or until the lentils and potatoes are tender.

1. Season to Taste:

- Once the lentils and vegetables are cooked through, season the soup with salt and pepper to taste, and adjust the seasoning as needed.

1. Serve:

- Remove the bay leaf from the soup before serving.
- Ladle the Lentil Soup with Carrots, Celery, and Potatoes into serving bowls.

• Garnish with fresh chopped parsley if desired.

• Serve hot with lemon wedges on the side for squeezing over the soup, if desired.

Nutrition Information (per serving):

• Calories: 250

• Protein: 15g

• Fat: 2g

• Carbohydrates: 45g

• Fiber: 12g

• Sugar: 5g

• Sodium: 800mg

BROWN RICE PILAF WITH PEAS AND CARROTS

Meal Description: This brown rice pilaf with peas and carrots is a wholesome and flavorful dish. It's a nutritious twist on a classic favorite that's perfect as a side dish or a light vegetarian meal. Nutty brown rice is cooked with aromatic onions, sweet peas, and tender carrots, creating a colorful and satisfying pilaf that's both delicious and comforting. Serve it alongside your favorite protein, or enjoy it on its own for a nourishing and satisfying meal.

Ingredients:

- 1 cup brown rice
- 2 cups vegetable or chicken broth
- One onion, finely chopped
- Two carrots diced
- 1 cup frozen peas
- Two cloves garlic, minced
- 2 tbsp olive oil
- 1 tsp dried thyme
- Salt and pepper to taste

• Fresh parsley for garnish (optional)

• Lemon wedges for serving (optional)

Instructions:

1. Cook Brown Rice:

• Rinse the brown rice under cold water until the water runs clear. Drain well.

• Heat olive oil in a large pot over medium heat. Add finely chopped onion and diced carrots. Sauté for 5-7 minutes or until the vegetables are softened.

1. Add Garlic and Rice:

• Add minced garlic to the pot and sauté for another minute until fragrant.

• Add the rinsed and drained brown rice to the pot. Stir to coat the rice with the vegetables and oil.

1. Simmer with Broth:

• Pour vegetable or chicken broth into the pot, along with dried thyme, salt, and pepper to taste. Stir to combine.

• Bring the mixture to a boil, then reduce the heat to low. Cover and simmer for 40-45 minutes or until the rice is tender and the liquid is absorbed.

1. Add Peas:

• Once the rice is cooked, add frozen peas to the pot. Stir to combine.

• Cover the pot and let it sit for a few minutes, allowing the residual heat to thaw and warm the peas.

1. Serve:

• Fluff the Brown Rice Pilaf with Peas and Carrots with a fork.

- Garnish with fresh chopped parsley if desired.

- Serve hot with lemon wedges on the side for squeezing over the pilaf, if desired.

Nutrition Information (per serving):

- Calories: 200

- Protein: 5g

- Fat: 5g

- Carbohydrates: 35g

- Fiber: 5g

- Sugar: 5g

- Sodium: 500mg

WHOLE GRAIN WRAP WITH TURKEY, CHEESE, LETTUCE, AND TOMATO

Meal Description: Satisfy your hunger with this delicious and nutritious Whole Grain Wrap with Turkey, Cheese, Lettuce, and Tomato—a wholesome and convenient meal that's perfect for lunch on the go or a quick dinner. Packed with lean protein, fiber-rich grains, and fresh vegetables, this flavorful wrap offers a balanced combination of flavors and textures that will keep you feeling satisfied and energized throughout the day.

Ingredients:

• One whole-grain wrap or tortilla

• Three slices of turkey breast

• One slice of cheese (such as cheddar, Swiss, or pepper jack)

• 1/4 cup shredded lettuce

• One slice of tomato

• Mustard or mayonnaise (optional)

• Salt and pepper to taste

Instructions:

1. Prepare Wrap:

• Lay the whole-grain wrap or tortilla on a clean, flat surface.

1. Layer Ingredients:

• Place the slices of turkey breast in the center of the wrap, leaving some space around the edges.

• Add a slice of cheese on top of the turkey.

1. Add Lettuce and Tomato:

• Arrange shredded lettuce evenly over the cheese.

• Place a slice of tomato on top of the lettuce.

1. Season and Optional Condiments:

• Season with salt and pepper to taste.

• If desired, spread a thin layer of mustard or mayonnaise over the turkey before adding the lettuce and tomato.

1. Wrap It Up:

• Fold the sides of the wrap towards the center, then roll it up tightly from the bottom, enclosing the filling.

• Press gently to seal the edges of the wrap.

1. Serve:

• Slice the Whole Grain Wrap with Turkey, Cheese, Lettuce, and Tomato in half diagonally or leave it whole.

• Serve immediately, or wrap it in parchment paper or foil for a convenient meal on the go.

Nutrition Information (per serving):

- Calories: 300
- Protein: 20g
- Fat: 10g
- Carbohydrates: 30g
- Fiber: 5g
- Sugar: 3g
- Sodium: 600mg

BULGUR SALAD WITH CHICKPEAS, CUCUMBER, AND FETA

Meal Description: Indulge in the delightful flavors and textures of this refreshing Bulgur Salad with Chickpeas, Cucumber, and Feta—a nutritious and satisfying dish that's perfect for lunch or as a side for dinner. Nutty bulgur wheat is paired with protein-packed chickpeas, crisp cucumber, tangy feta cheese, and aromatic herbs tossed in a zesty lemon vinaigrette. Whether enjoyed on its own or as a complement to grilled meats or fish, this vibrant salad is sure to tantalize your taste buds and leave you feeling nourished and satisfied.

Ingredients:

For the Salad:

- 1 cup bulgur wheat

- One can (15 oz) chickpeas, drained and rinsed

- One cucumber, diced

- 1/2 cup crumbled feta cheese

- 1/4 cup chopped fresh parsley

- 2 tbsp chopped fresh mint

- Salt and pepper to taste

For the Lemon Vinaigrette:

- 1/4 cup extra virgin olive oil

- 2 tbsp freshly squeezed lemon juice

- 1 tsp Dijon mustard

- One clove of garlic, minced

- Salt and pepper to taste

Instructions:

1. Cook Bulgur Wheat:

- In a medium saucepan, bring 2 cups of water to a boil. Add bulgur wheat to the boiling water and stir.

- Reduce the heat to low, cover, and simmer for 10-12 minutes or until the bulgur is tender and the water is absorbed.

- Remove from heat and let it cool slightly.

1. Prepare Lemon Vinaigrette:

- In a small bowl, whisk together extra virgin olive oil, freshly squeezed lemon juice, Dijon mustard, minced garlic, salt, and pepper until well combined.

1. Assemble Salad:

- In a large mixing bowl, combine cooked bulgur wheat, drained and rinsed chickpeas, diced cucumber, crumbled feta cheese, chopped fresh parsley, and chopped fresh mint.

- Pour the prepared lemon vinaigrette over the salad ingredients.

1. Toss and Season:

• Gently toss the salad until all ingredients are evenly coated with the dressing.

• Season with salt and pepper to taste.

1. Chill and Serve:

• Cover the Bulgur Salad with Chickpeas, Cucumber, and Feta and refrigerate for at least 30 minutes to allow the flavors to meld.

• Before serving, taste and adjust seasoning if necessary.

• Serve chilled or at room temperature, garnished with additional fresh herbs if desired.

Nutrition Information (per serving):

• Calories: 300

• Protein: 10g

• Fat: 15g

• Carbohydrates: 35g

• Fiber: 8g

• Sugar: 3g

• Sodium: 400mg

CHAPTER SIX

Hydration Recipes

Infused Water with Cucumber, Mint, and Lemon

Beverage Description: Stay refreshed and hydrated with this invigorating Infused Water with Cucumber, Mint, and Lemon—a delightful and healthy alternative to sugary drinks. Fresh cucumber slices, fragrant mint leaves, and zesty lemon slices are combined in cold Water, infusing it with subtle flavors and a refreshing aroma. Enjoy this hydrating beverage any time of the day for a burst of natural flavor and a revitalizing boost.

Ingredients:

• 1/2 cucumber, thinly sliced

• 5-6 fresh mint leaves

• 1/2 lemon, thinly sliced

• 6 cups cold Water

• Ice cubes (optional)

Instructions:

1. Prepare Ingredients:

• Wash the cucumber, mint leaves, and lemon in cold Water.

• Thinly slice the cucumber and lemon.

• Gently crush the mint leaves to release their aroma.

1. Combine Ingredients:

• Add the thinly sliced cucumber, crushed mint leaves, and lemon slices in a large pitcher or glass jar.

1. Add Water:

• Pour cold Water into the pitcher or jar, completely

covering the cucumber, mint, and lemon slices.

1. Infuse:

• Stir the ingredients gently to distribute the flavors.

• Cover the pitcher or jar and refrigerate for at least 1-2 hours or overnight for more robust flavor.

1. Serve:

• When ready to serve, give the infused Water a final stir.

• If desired, fill glasses with ice cubes and pour the infused Water over the ice.

• Garnish each glass with a cucumber slice, mint leaf, or lemon slice for an extra touch of freshness.

1. Enjoy:

• Sip and enjoy Infused Water's calm and refreshing taste with Cucumber, Mint, and Lemon.

• Refill the pitcher with Water as needed to continue enjoying infused Water throughout the day.

Note: Feel free to customize this infused water recipe by adjusting the quantities of cucumber, mint, and lemon to suit your taste preferences. For different flavor variations, you can also experiment with other additions, such as sliced strawberries, orange slices, or ginger.

Iced Green Tea with Fresh Lime

Beverage Description: Quench your thirst and invigorate your senses with this revitalizing Iced Green Tea with Fresh Lime—a refreshing and antioxidant-rich drink that's perfect for any time of day. Fragrant green tea is brewed and chilled, then infused with the bright zestiness of fresh lime juice, creating a vibrant and uplifting beverage that's both cooling and invigorating.

Sip on this flavorful concoction to stay hydrated and energized throughout the day.

Ingredients:

• Four green tea bags

• 6 cups Water

• 2-3 fresh limes, juiced

• Ice cubes

• Fresh lime slices for garnish (optional)

• Honey or sweetener of choice (optional)

Instructions:

1. Brew Green Tea:

• Bring 6 cups of Water to a large pot or kettle boil.

• Remove from heat and add green tea bags to the hot Water.

• Allow the tea bags to steep for 3-5 minutes, depending on desired strength.

1. Chill Tea:

• Once brewed, remove the tea bags from the pot and discard them.

• Let the brewed green tea cool to room temperature, then transfer it to the refrigerator to chill for at least 1 hour.

1. Prepare Limes:

• While the tea is chilling, juice the fresh limes to extract the juice.

• You can also slice some lime wedges for garnish if desired.

1. Assemble Drink:

• Combine the chilled green tea with the freshly squeezed lime juice in a large pitcher.

• Stir well to mix the flavors.

1. Serve:

• Fill glasses with ice cubes.

• Pour the Iced Green Tea with Fresh Lime into the glasses.

• Garnish each glass with a slice of fresh lime, if desired.

1. Sweeten (Optional):

• If you prefer a sweeter taste, you can add honey or your preferred sweetener to the iced tea and stir until dissolved.

1. Enjoy:

• Sip and enjoy the excellent, refreshing taste of Iced Green Tea with Fresh Lime.

• Store any remaining tea in the refrigerator and consume it within a few days for optimal freshness.

Note: Feel free to adjust the amount of lime juice according to your taste preference. For extra freshness and complexity, you can add additional flavorings, such as fresh mint leaves or slices of cucumber.

COCONUT WATER SMOOTHIE WITH PINEAPPLE AND SPINACH

Beverage Description: Energize your day with this vibrant and nutritious Coconut Water Smoothie with Pineapple and Spinach. It's a refreshing blend of tropical flavors and leafy greens that's sure to leave you feeling rejuvenated. Sweet pineapple adds a burst of tropical sweetness, while fresh spinach provides a dose of green goodness. Combined with hydrating coconut water, this smoothie is delicious, hydrating, and packed with vitamins and minerals. Sip on this revitalizing beverage for a refreshing start to your day or a midday pick-me-up.

Ingredients:

• 1 cup coconut water

• 1 cup fresh or frozen pineapple chunks

• 1 cup fresh spinach leaves

• 1/2 banana, frozen (optional for added creaminess)

• 1/2 cup ice cubes (if not using frozen pineapple or banana)

• Honey or maple syrup (optional for sweetness)

Instructions:

1. Prepare Ingredients:

• If using fresh pineapple, peel and cut it into chunks.

• If not using a frozen banana, peel and slice the banana into chunks and freeze them beforehand.

1. Blend Smoothie:

• In a blender, combine the coconut water, pineapple chunks, fresh spinach leaves, and frozen banana (if using).

• Add ice cubes to the blender to chill and thicken the smoothie if not using a frozen banana.

1. Blend Until Smooth:

• Blend the ingredients on high speed until smooth and creamy.

• If the smoothie is too thick, you can add more coconut water to reach your desired consistency.

1. Adjust Sweetness (Optional):

• Taste the smoothie and add honey or maple syrup if desired for additional sweetness.

• Blend again briefly to incorporate the sweetener.

1. Serve:

• Pour the Coconut Water Smoothie with Pineapple and Spinach into glasses.

• Garnish with a pineapple wedge or a sprinkle of shredded coconut if desired.

1. Enjoy:

• Sip and enjoy the tropical flavors and nourishing goodness of this refreshing smoothie.

• Serve immediately for the best taste and texture.

Note: Feel free to customize this smoothie recipe by adding other fruits or ingredients such as mango, kiwi, avocado, or protein powder for an extra boost. Adjust the quantities of ingredients to suit your taste preferences and dietary needs.

SPARKLING WATER WITH FRESH BERRIES AND MINT

Beverage Description: Elevate your hydration game with this refreshing Sparkling Water with Fresh Berries and Mint—a bubbly and invigorating drink that's as visually stunning as it is delicious. Vibrant mixed berries add a burst of natural sweetness and vibrant color, while fresh mint leaves provide a cool and refreshing aroma. Combined with crisp and effervescent sparkling Water, this beverage is a perfect way to stay hydrated and refreshed on a hot day or as a delightful accompaniment to any meal.

Ingredients:

• 1 cup mixed fresh berries (such as strawberries, blueberries, raspberries, and blackberries)

• Fresh mint leaves

• Sparkling Water (plain or flavored, as desired)

• Ice cubes

Instructions:

1. Prepare Ingredients:

• Wash the mixed berries and pat them dry with a paper

towel.

• Remove any stems or hulls from the berries as needed.

• Rinse the fresh mint leaves under cold Water and pat them dry.

1. Muddle Berries and Mint:

• Add a handful of mixed berries and a few fresh mint leaves in a tall glass or pitcher.

• Use a muddler or the back of a spoon to gently crush and muddle the berries and mint leaves, releasing their flavors and juices.

1. Add Ice:

• Fill the glass with ice cubes to chill the drink and keep it refreshing.

1. Pour Sparkling Water:

• Pour sparkling Water into the glass over the muddled berries, mint, and ice cubes. For added variety, use plain sparkling Water or flavored sparkling Water.

1. Stir:

• Use a long spoon or straw to gently stir the ingredients together, distributing the flavors throughout the sparkling Water.

1. Garnish:

• Garnish the drink with additional fresh berries and mint leaves for a beautiful presentation.

1. Serve:

• Serve the Sparkling Water with Fresh Berries and Mint immediately, and enjoy its effervescent, fruity, and refreshing taste.

Note: Feel free to customize this beverage by using your favorite berry combination or adding other fruits, such as citrus slices or cucumber, for extra flavor. If desired, adjust the sweetness by adding a drizzle of honey or agave syrup.

HERBAL TEA WITH GINGER AND LEMON

Beverage Description: Soothe your senses and invigorate your spirit with this comforting Herbal Tea with Ginger and Lemon—a warming and aromatic infusion that's perfect for relaxing moments or as a natural remedy for colds and sore throats. Fragrant ginger root adds a spicy kick and soothing warmth, while fresh lemon slices impart a bright and citrusy flavor. Whether enjoyed hot on a chilly day or chilled over ice for a refreshing twist, this herbal tea is sure to delight your taste buds and nourish your body.

Ingredients:

• 2 cups Water

• 1-inch piece of fresh ginger, thinly sliced

• One lemon, thinly sliced

• Honey or agave syrup (optional for sweetness)

Instructions:

1. Prepare Ingredients:

• Rinse the fresh ginger under cold Water to remove any dirt.

• Use a sharp knife or vegetable peeler to thinly slice the ginger.

• Rinse the lemon under cold Water and slice it thinly.

1. Boil Water:

• Bring 2 cups of Water to a boil over medium heat in a small saucepan.

1. Infuse Ginger:

• Once the Water is boiling, add the thinly sliced ginger to the saucepan.

• Reduce the heat to low and let the ginger simmer in the Water for 5-7 minutes to infuse its flavor.

1. Add Lemon:

• After simmering the ginger, add the thinly sliced lemon to the saucepan.

• Let the lemon slices simmer with the ginger-infused Water for an additional 2-3 minutes.

1. Remove from Heat:

• Remove the saucepan from the heat once the ginger and lemon have infused their flavors into the Water.

1. Strain and Serve:

• Use a fine-mesh sieve or tea strainer to strain the herbal tea, removing the ginger and lemon slices.

• Pour the strained tea into cups or mugs for serving.

1. Sweeten (Optional):

• If desired, add honey or agave syrup to sweeten the tea to taste. Stir until the sweetener is dissolved.

1. Serve Hot or Cold:

• Serve the Herbal Tea with Ginger and Lemon hot for a comforting drink, or let it cool and serve it chilled over ice for a refreshing beverage.

Note: You can adjust the strength of the tea by steeping the ginger and lemon for longer or shorter periods of time, depending on your preference for flavor intensity. You can also experiment with adding other herbs or spices, such as mint or cinnamon, for additional depth of flavor.

FRUIT-INFUSED WATER WITH WATERMELON AND BASIL

Beverage Description: Indulge in the refreshing and revitalizing flavors of this Fruit-Infused Water with Watermelon and Basil. This delightful and hydrating drink is perfect for hot summer days or any time you need a cooling pick-me-up. Juicy watermelon chunks lend a subtle sweetness and refreshing juiciness, while fresh basil leaves add a touch of herbal aroma and complexity. Sip on this infused Water for a burst of natural flavor and a rejuvenating boost to your day.

Ingredients:

• 4 cups cold Water

• 2 cups seedless watermelon, cubed

• Handful of fresh basil leaves

• Ice cubes (optional)

Instructions:

1. Prepare Ingredients:

• Wash the watermelon thoroughly under cold Water.

• Cut the watermelon into small cubes, discarding any seeds.

• Rinse the fresh basil leaves under cold Water and pat them dry with a paper towel.

1. Combine Ingredients:

• Add the cubed watermelon and fresh basil leaves in a large pitcher or glass jar.

1. Mash Ingredients:

• Use a muddler or the back of a spoon to mash the watermelon and basil together in the pitcher gently. This will help release their flavors.

1. Add Water:

• Pour cold Water into the pitcher, covering the mashed watermelon and basil completely.

1. Chill:

• Place the pitcher in the refrigerator and let the fruit-infused water chill for at least 1 hour to allow the flavors to meld.

1. Serve:

• When ready to serve, fill glasses with ice cubes if desired.

• Pour the Fruit-Infused Water with Watermelon and Basil into glasses, making sure to distribute the watermelon and basil evenly.

1. Garnish (Optional):

• For an extra touch of freshness and presentation, garnish each glass with a sprig of fresh basil or a watermelon wedge.

1. Enjoy:

• Sip and enjoy the crisp and refreshing taste of this Fruit-Infused Water with Watermelon and Basil as a hydrating and rejuvenating beverage.

Note: Feel free to customize this infused water recipe by adding other fruits or herbs, such as cucumber, mint, or lime, for different flavor variations. If desired, adjust the sweetness by adding a drizzle of honey or agave syrup.

ELECTROLYTE DRINK WITH COCONUT WATER, LIME, AND SEA SALT

Beverage Description: Rehydrate and replenish your body with this revitalizing Electrolyte Drink with Coconut Water, Lime, and Sea Salt. It's a natural and refreshing beverage perfect for post-workout recovery or staying hydrated on hot days. Nutrient-rich coconut water serves as the base, providing essential electrolytes like potassium and magnesium, while fresh lime juice adds a zesty citrus flavor. A pinch of sea salt enhances the drink with additional electrolytes, making it a hydrating and replenishing beverage that's both delicious and beneficial for overall well-being.

Ingredients:

• 2 cups coconut water

• Juice of 1 lime

• Pinch of sea salt

• Ice cubes (optional)

Instructions:

1. Prepare Ingredients:

• Squeeze the juice of one lime into a small bowl or cup.

• Measure out the coconut water and sea salt.

1. Combine Ingredients:

• In a large glass or pitcher, pour the coconut water.

• Add the freshly squeezed lime juice to the coconut water.

1. Add Sea Salt:

• Sprinkle a pinch of sea salt into the coconut water and lime mixture. The sea salt will help replenish electrolytes lost through sweating.

1. Stir Well:

• Use a spoon to stir the ingredients together until the sea salt is dissolved.

1. Chill (Optional):

• Place the Electrolyte Drink with Coconut Water, Lime, and Sea Salt in the refrigerator to chill for a refreshing cold beverage.

1. Serve:

• Fill glasses with ice cubes if desired.

• Pour the prepared electrolyte drink into glasses for serving.

1. Garnish (Optional):

• Garnish each glass with a slice of lime or a sprig of fresh mint for a decorative touch.

1. Enjoy:

• Sip and enjoy this Electrolyte Drink's crisp and refreshing taste, made with Coconut Water, Lime, and

Sea Salt, as a hydrating and revitalizing beverage.

Note: Feel free to adjust the lime juice and sea salt amount according to your taste preferences. You can also add a touch of honey or agave syrup for sweetness if desired.

HOMEMADE LEMONADE WITH STEVIA OR HONEY

Beverage Description: Quench your thirst with this classic Homemade Lemonade with Stevia or Honey—a refreshing and tangy drink perfect for sunny days or whenever you need an excellent and revitalizing pick-me-up. Freshly squeezed lemon juice provides a burst of citrus flavor, while sweet stevia or honey adds just the right amount of sweetness to balance the tartness. Served over ice, this homemade lemonade will be a hit with friends and family alike, making it a staple for summer gatherings or a refreshing treat any time of year.

Ingredients:

- 1 cup freshly squeezed lemon juice (about 4-6 lemons)

- 4 cups cold Water

- 1/4 - 1/2 cup stevia or honey (adjust to taste)

- Ice cubes

- Lemon slices for garnish (optional)

- Fresh mint leaves for garnish (optional)

Instructions:

1. Prepare Ingredients:

• Squeeze fresh lemon juice from the lemons, removing any seeds. You should have about 1 cup of lemon juice.

1. Mix Lemonade:

• Combine the freshly squeezed lemon juice with cold Water in a large pitcher.

• Stir well to mix the lemon juice and Water together.

1. Sweeten:

• Add stevia or honey to the pitcher, starting with 1/4 cup and adjusting to taste.

• Stir the lemonade well to dissolve the sweetener completely.

1. Taste and Adjust:

• Taste the lemonade and adjust the sweetness by adding more stevia or honey if desired.

1. Chill:

• Place the pitcher of Homemade Lemonade in the refrigerator to chill for at least 30 minutes before serving.

1. Serve:

• Fill glasses with ice cubes.

• Pour the chilled Homemade Lemonade into glasses.

1. Garnish (Optional):

• Garnish each glass with a slice of lemon and a sprig of fresh mint for an extra touch of freshness and presentation.

1. Enjoy:

• Sip and enjoy the crisp and tangy flavor of Homemade

Lemonade with Stevia or Honey as a refreshing and revitalizing beverage.

Note: Feel free to adjust the amount of stevia or honey according to your taste preferences. For additional complexity, you can experiment with adding other flavorings, such as fresh berries or herbs. Adjust the sweetness and tartness to suit your taste.

CONCLUSION

In conclusion, the metabolic confusion diet presents a novel approach to weight management by advocating for the strategic manipulation of dietary variables to keep the metabolism dynamic and responsive. While the concept holds promise in theory, its efficacy and long-term sustainability warrant further investigation. Proponents argue that individuals can prevent metabolic adaptation, stimulate fat loss, and support overall metabolic health by constantly varying aspects of one's diet, such as calorie intake, macronutrient composition, and meal timing.

However, this approach's lack of robust empirical evidence and potential risks underscores the need for caution. Critics contend that metabolic confusion may promote unhealthy eating habits, lead to nutritional imbalances, and lack the scientific substantiation needed to justify widespread adoption. Moreover, individual responses to these strategies can vary significantly, highlighting the importance of personalized approaches and close supervision by qualified healthcare professionals.

Despite these challenges, metabolic confusion prompts important discussions about the complexities of human metabolism and the potential impact of dietary interventions on metabolic health. Moving forward, continued research efforts are necessary to elucidate the mechanisms underlying metabolic confusion and determine its efficacy, safety, and feasibility as a long-term strategy for weight management.

In the interim, individuals seeking to optimize their metabolic health and achieve sustainable weight loss are encouraged to focus on evidence-based principles such as consuming a balanced diet rich in whole foods, engaging in regular physical activity, and prioritizing overall well-being. By embracing a holistic approach to health and wellness, individuals can cultivate lifelong habits that support metabolic health and promote lasting success in achieving their health and fitness goals.